Praise for Dr. Blaich's *Your Inner Pharmacy*

"Dr. Blaich addresses in a clear voice the wisdom of the mind-body in the creation of health."
—Amy Mills, M.D. Diplomat, American Board of Psychiatry and Neurology and American Board of Holistic Medicine

"*Your Inner Pharmacy* will assist many people to understand how to retrieve and enhance their capacity to deal with change and stress and enable them to function in a way that is required for the exciting competitive lifestyle that almost all Americans will face for the rest of their lives. The book is not only something to be read from cover to cover but will serve as a long-term resource as they encounter more and more challenges including how to age wisely and remain productive."
—Christopher J. Hegarty, Ph.D., author, researcher, and public speaker

"I have been a competitive athlete for over thirty-five years. Yet at no time have I experienced better overall health, fitness, and balance than in this past year of working with Dr. Blaich. With his knowledge, patience, expertise, and healing hands, he has helped me attain the priceless state of integrated well-being, which has contributed to athletic achievement I never expected. A huge thank you to Dr. Blaich."
—Ellen Hart Pena, public speaker, attorney, and Olympic trials participant

"There are billions of words written on health and healthcare. Where can health consumers possibly get their heads around the subject? The answer is here in Dr. Blaich's masterfully written, well-organized, and well-illustrated book. A rare and fortunate find for today's bewildered healthcare consumer."
—Scott Walker, D.C., founder of NeuroEmotional Technique

"Robert Blaich has written a book about health—the real meaning of it—and about aging. He is worth everyone's time, even if, like me, one is a doubter. Unlike people with miracle diets or theories to fix parts of your life, Dr. Blaich shows us a total picture of how to live, making the most of what we have been given and balancing that with what we can do to minimize our individual shortcomings—those things that define us as much as our strengths do.... Every time I stand before an orchestra and give an upbeat, I thank Robert Blaich. No matter what you do in your life, I believe you will thank him too."

—**John Mauceri**, conductor of the Hollywood Bowl Orchestra

"This book will benefit anyone interested in more good years of life, and that is all of us. Dr. Blaich's clear and interesting storytelling of the latest scientific evidence for natural and complementary approaches will hold your interest and change your life for the better."

—**John F. Thie, D.C.**, founder of Touch for Health

"One of the great memories I have of Bob is when he cautiously intruded into my life and invited himself to be my personal physician at the 1984 Olympic games. Looking back, I know that without his support, that day I won the gold would not have ended with the success that it did."

—**Alexi Grewal**, Olympic Gold Medalist in men's cycling

"Dr. Blaich has presented a tremendous amount of material in *Your Inner Pharmacy* and explained it in a way that the average person can understand. I will definitely recommend this book to all my patients so that they can make more informed choices in deciding their healthcare options."

—**James M. Kennedy, D.D.S.**, former president of the Holistic Dental Association

Your Inner Pharmacy

Congratulations!
You now own an Enhanced Book.™
There is more content than fits between its covers.
Registration is free.
More pages, photos, updates, and information are included.
Just log onto the URL below and enjoy!

Your **free enhanced version**
of this book is at
www.enhancedbooks.com!

158☐270☐14☐58

Your Inner Pharmacy

taking back our wellness

DR. ROBERT BLAICH

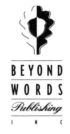

BEYOND
WORDS
Publishing
I N C

Beyond Words Publishing, Inc.
20827 N.W. Cornell Road, Suite 500
Hillsboro, Oregon 97124-9808
503-531-8700
503-531-8773 fax
www.beyondword.com

The information contained in this book is intended to be educational and not for diagnosis, prescription, or treatment of any health disorder whatsoever. This information should not replace consultation with a competent healthcare professional. The content of the book is intended to be used as an adjunct to a rational and responsible healthcare program prescribed by a professional healthcare practitioner. The author and publisher are in no way liable for any use or misuse of the material.

Editor: Laura O. Foster
Managing editor: Henry Covey
Proofreader: Marvin Moore
Cover and interior design: Carol Sibley
Composition: William H. Brunson Typography Services

Printed in the United States of America
Library of Congress Cataloging-in-Publication Data
Blaich, Robert.
    Your inner pharmacy : taking back our wellness / Robert Blaich.
        p. cm.
    Includes bibliographical references and index.
    ISBN-13: 978-1-58270-145-5 (hardcover : alk. paper)
    1. Self-care, Health.   2. Integrative medicine.   3. Health.   I. Title.
RA776.95.B53   2005
613—dc22

                                                        2005037794

The corporate mission of Beyond Words Publishing, Inc.:
    Inspire to Integrity

To Lindell, Megan, and Bonnie

CONTENTS

ACKNOWLEDGMENTS

The first thanks go to my parents, Dorothy and Merrill, and to my sister, Carol, who created a wonderfully supportive, stimulating, and diverse environment for me to grow up in.

I have also been extremely fortunate to have so many great teachers along the way. After graduate school, my patients, students, and colleagues became my teachers. I am very thankful for all the patients I have treated and the thousands of doctors who have attended my seminars over the years. You have inspired me to learn more deeply and to explain more clearly.

Thank you, Dr. George Goodheart, for your brilliant observations and insatiable curiosity, which led to the creation and development of Applied Kinesiology.

Getting a book started presents a challenge, and I thank my friend Bill Sumner for his motivation. Dr. Richard Gardella was also very helpful with his early editorial assistance. David Kropf provided editing and guidance, over several years, which helped immensely in the development of this book. A special thanks goes to Parker Collier for her encouragement and support in this project.

Many people read my manuscript at various stages and provided feedback and ideas for its further development. Peter Kreitler, Andy Leonard, Alan Santos, John Mauceri, Pete Douglas, Esther Nichols,

Acknowledgments

Tom Dietvorst, George Goodheart, Alex Ediss, Walter Schmitt, and Scott Varley provided especially valuable input. Thanks also to my colleague Dr. Scott Monk, who worked with me in creating the graphics.

Thank you, Christopher Hegarty, for believing in me and for introducing me to Beyond Words Publishing. Cynthia Black and the whole team at Beyond Words have been wonderful to work with.

A very special acknowledgment goes to my wife, Lindell, and our daughters, Megan and Bonnie. You all bring so much beauty, joy, and love into my life.

INTRODUCTION

The healthcare landscape has changed. Breakthrough solutions in the nineteenth and twentieth centuries controlled the spread of acute and infectious diseases and provided people with greater life spans. But today, technologically advanced countries face different challenges to health, one of which is an enormous increase in chronic diseases such as cardiovascular disease, arthritis, and Type 2 diabetes. What worked so well in the treatment of acute and infectious disease simply doesn't work for chronic disease. And unfortunately, what most people—doctors and patients—have not yet recognized is that we are treating individuals for their symptoms without addressing the source of the ill health. Truly, much of chronic disease is self-inflicted—a result of how you and I live and how we look at health and disease. *Your Inner Pharmacy* looks at this problem and shows you how you can avoid or minimize the effects of chronic illness by improving your health.

The trend toward more and earlier occurrences of chronic disease means lost years and a declining quality of life that compromises many of us from middle age into our final decades. The core of the problem truly is how we look at health and disease. The good news is that this core contains the seeds for new solutions. The solution lies in our deeply ingrained attitudes. When we change the way we look at health and disease, our priorities change. The action steps that we can take to improve our health and decrease the deterioration of our bodies happen naturally when we hold a deep-seated understanding of what is at stake and what can be gained through a proactive approach. Unfortunately, the sea of information and misinformation about health and disease has led most of us to not know where to begin to sort it out, to not know what questions to ask or even who to ask them to.

Here it is in a nutshell. In a typical lifespan, you rapidly move from the "invincibility of youth" to the onset of chronic disease. Health is taken for granted until it is lost. And our automatic response is to turn first to medications to control symptoms. We have come to expect that it is normal to take one or more lifelong medications beginning at an early age. The focus on disease and on controlling symptoms has clearly become "Plan A." Within this scenario, degenerative disease is increasing and healthcare costs are spiraling out of control. Baby boomers as well as their children and grandchildren are missing out on opportunities for vitality in their lives and quality time together.

Great technological and pharmacological advances over the past century have provided us with more years to live. Yet when combined with stressful lifestyles and deteriorating diets, these extra years also provide more opportunity for the advancement of chronic disease, which all too often removes the quality of life from those years so nicely added on at the end.

The great progress made in the treatment of acute and infectious diseases is being overshadowed by the enormous increase in chronic diseases such as osteoarthritis, GERD, asthma, heart disease, elevated blood pressure, diabetes, and anxiety/depression or mood disorders. Standard first line of treatment is to use medications to control them. However, unlike infectious diseases, where the right medication solved the problem by killing off the invading agent, chronic diseases are rarely caused by outside invaders. Rather, they are caused by malfunctions within the body itself and are not eliminated by a "one size fits all" approach.

Chronic diseases do, fortunately, often respond to treatments that normalize and improve the function of the body. The fact is that you have a pharmacy within your body—your Inner Pharmacy—that creates many good and bad chemicals. Moreover, you were born with a body that has a phenomenal ability to regulate and heal itself. Restoring and promoting its normal function should be the first line of treatment for most ongoing, low-grade, non-life-threatening problems, otherwise known as chronic disease.

Given the opportunity, your Inner Pharmacy can keep you healthy and ward off chronic disease for a lifetime. A properly functioning body and a healthy lifestyle combine to maintain and sustain the normal function of your body so that it requires less outside intervention throughout life.

The external pharmacy—drugs, both prescribed and over the counter—provide man-made chemicals to the body from the outside, and they should be the first line of treatment only for emergencies, acute situations, and advanced disease, when it is necessary to regulate and replace what the body can no longer do on its own.

It is not my intention to criticize mainstream Western medicine, which prolongs and saves many lives. I do hope to show you that other healthcare options exist, both complementary and alternative, especially in the realm of chronic disease. When you recognize that most chronic disease is not an illness you "get" but rather a set of symptoms that result from the body's failure to regulate itself, you can understand how chronic disease—whether it is arthritis or gastritis—will not be eradicated by medications. When you treat your chronic condition only with medications that control symptoms, your body's underlying malfunctions can continue to worsen and the "disease" advances, despite the illusion that you are improving. The ideal treatment would work not only to control symptoms but also to correct the underlying malfunctions that are creating them. It makes no sense to ignore the power of the Inner Pharmacy.

I am not anti-drug. I am pro-health. What I am suggesting is an approach to your health that actually improves your body's function. It is logical, systematic, and straightforward, and it can be implemented immediately. It is comprehensive and yet simple. It's just different from the way we have been taught to think. The only challenging part is that understanding its significance and value may require a shift in your perspective. But once you see how much we have all missed the obvious, you will want to create and begin living your own health plan. It's a matter of making health a priority, of creating health, which creates quality time—which is what everyone wants. Using your Inner Pharmacy to create health not only improves your productivity, performance, and quality of life now, but it also goes a long way toward delaying and preventing the onset of chronic disease.

Like any doctor, I can tell you how to take care of many specific problems, and I can tell you steps to take to improve your health. I'm perfectly willing to do that, but it still makes you dependent on me to solve problems for you. As a healthcare provider, I'd really rather guide you to creating for yourself a richer, fuller life, one in which you have fewer problems to begin with and can solve more of them on your own when they do arise. That is not to say that you should ignore professional help for any health problem; it is merely to say that if you understand and follow certain principles, you will have less need for outside intervention from a healthcare system whose current focus is on treating sickness, illness, and disease rather than on creating health.

Part 1 of this book looks at the healthcare crisis and sheds light on the core of the healthcare system's failure: a set of cultural attitudes about health and the responsibility for your health, my health, or your child's health. Once we recognize these attitudes, it's not hard to change them and to consider healthcare in a way that empowers us to take charge of our own health.

Part 2 looks at the enormous difference between treating a symptom and treating the person who has the symptom. The former is the traditional Western model; the latter is the holistic healthcare approach. This section tells a story of what goes on in a holistic practice, including the thought process of how health and restoring the normal function of the body are looked at and how some of the treatments are applied.

Part 2 also discusses the three major areas that impact your health: the raw materials you provide your body (diet and supplements); your lifestyle (including stress and how you handle it, and exercise); and a properly functioning body. Even with a perfect score on the first two items, you can compromise your health when you do not take advantage of the range of healthcare that restores the proper function of your body, especially after illness or injury. Since both of these alter your physiology and normal body function, they can precede chronic disease and may be the biggest single cause of advanced aging and premature degeneration. It's like never maintaining a car and wondering why it falls apart after thirty or fifty thousand miles. This book focuses on how to complement good eating and lifestyle habits with using good healthcare that addresses your own health needs—without resorting to a pill.

In nearly thirty years of treating patients in clinical practice, I have witnessed miraculous responses that occur when the body is restored to its normal state of physiology. The return to health and the improvement in human performance occurs when the healing power of nature can do its work. It's not magical healing. On the contrary, identifying and correcting abnormal function in the body requires a deep understanding of practical science. It's the same science everyone uses; the only difference is the practical application of it to improve health, not just to treat disease.

Part 3 is the springboard to action: It's where you stop reading and start creating your own health. The formula is simple: Invest 10 percent of your weekly leisure time into health-promoting activities—and with a properly functioning body, the result will be health and the actual creation of quality time. With as little as five hours a week, you can delay the degeneration and decline in body function that compromises quality of life. Invest time to create time: It's no different from systematically investing money for your future needs. You'll need money in your old age; don't you want good health to go with it?

Make health a priority in your daily life. Use your Inner Pharmacy first. It's never too late to start, and the sooner the better. The benefits that accumulate for the future will also improve your health and performance now.

Part 1

The New Landscape

1

UNDERSTANDING CHRONIC DISEASE

Infectious diseases are no longer responsible for most of the world's deaths, and as of 2004, the world now has more overweight people (over 1 billion) than malnourished people (800 million), according to the World Health Organization.[1] In 2005, WHO acknowledged chronic disease as a "global epidemic" and estimated that of the 58 million total deaths that year, 35 million would be from chronic conditions.[2] In the United States, chronic disease is now the principal cause of disability, and it consumes 78 percent of the nation's health expenditures.[3] Let's look at what "chronic disease" means.

In the United States alone, more than 125 million people (almost one-third of the population) live with a chronic condition such as cardiovascular disease, arthritis, or type 2 diabetes. By 2020, the number will be an estimated 157 million.[4] You—along with your friends, family, and co-workers—are most likely headed toward chronic disease. If you live long enough, your health and quality of life will be compromised. Parts of your body will no longer function as they once did; they'll ache, break, or outright fail. It's depressing, but this is a fact of life and the essence of the aging process.

Now the good news, which is the focus of this book: Options exist, wonderful and realistic options that offer you more good years of life, perhaps five, ten, even twenty or more years of quality time. These options can postpone and often minimize the onset of chronic diseases. It requires only that you look at your health in a different way than you are accustomed to.

Your quality of life, now and for years to come, is a result of choices you make along the way. One of the most critical choices you can make is to shift away from an illness mentality, i.e., reacting to and fearing disease. Instead, shift your outlook to health; anticipate health and create your health—now.

Let's begin by looking at the nature of chronic disease and how it differs from acute disease.

From Dysfunction to Disease

Chronic disease develops gradually as a result of dysfunction in the body. This is not something that our culture teaches us. But arthritis, hypertension, gastroesophageal reflux disease (commonly known as GERD), type 2 diabetes, coronary heart disease, and even many cancers are not diseases that people suddenly "get." They are each preceded by years of dysfunction in the body, involving a gradual deterioration of normal function over time. Once deterioration reaches a certain level, it becomes recognizable as disease. Rather than *get* a chronic disease, we *develop* or *acquire* it when our lifestyle activates or triggers genetic predispositions for weaknesses in specific areas. At some point then, our body loses its native ability to regulate itself and then requires outside intervention.

This process is quite different from an acute disease such as tuberculosis, which a person does, in fact, "get" if it is transmitted to the body by specific bacteria that the immune system is unable to ward off. Antibiotics have made great strides at minimizing or eliminating acute and infectious diseases, particularly those of a bacterial nature.

When suffering from an acute disease, you, as patient, can be passive and uninformed, since usually only one potential treatment option exists. Essentially, it is the disease that is treated, not you. The acute disease is typically a brief episode followed, ideally, by a cure, in which you return to normal or pre-disease status.

4

In chronic disease, however, your role as patient is drastically different. First, chronic diseases are rarely cured. Instead, they are managed, as a continuous, ongoing process in which you, as patient, eventually become actively involved out of necessity. During the years after diagnosis, choices often exist for both treatment and lifestyle modifications, which directly affect the disease progression. In chronic disease, the physician does more *with* the patient rather than *to* his disease. The physician shares some responsibility and decision making with the patient and takes on the additional roles of teacher and even coach.

If you suffer a chronic disease, you do not need to resign yourself to an eventual downhill slide. You can educate yourself as to what malfunctions in your body cause the disease to occur and to advance. You can then work to improve those functions to prevent further deterioration and perhaps restore some of the normal function that has been lost. With chronic disease, knowledgeable patients achieve better outcomes. Parts 2 and 3 of this book will guide you to more effective healthcare and to the creation of a healthier lifestyle for yourself.

A genetic weak link that has been continually triggered by inappropriate diet or a stressful lifestyle eventually becomes a disease. In other words, dysfunction progresses into disease. Figure 1 illustrates this concept.

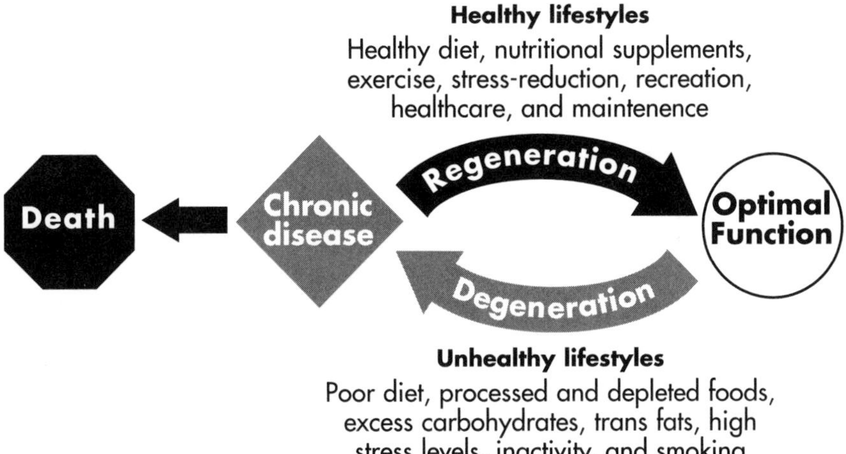

Healthy lifestyles
Healthy diet, nutritional supplements,
exercise, stress-reduction, recreation,
healthcare, and maintenence

Death ← Chronic disease — Regeneration → Optimal Function

Degeneration

Unhealthy lifestyles
Poor diet, processed and depleted foods,
excess carbohydrates, trans fats, high
stress levels, inactivity, and smoking

Figure 1

Healthy lifestyles shift this continuum toward normal—or even optimal—function. A healthy lifestyle includes aerobic exercise, stress-reducing recreation, a healthful diet with nutritional supplements, and healthcare that strengthens the weak links in your body. Each healthy lifestyle factor has a cumulative effect toward promoting normal function in the body. Unhealthy lifestyles all shift the continuum toward degeneration and death. An unhealthy lifestyle is one that is quite common in technologically advanced nations: consumption of trans fats and excess carbohydrates, diets devoid of adequate nutrients, sedentary existence, high stress levels, and smoking.

Because you have the power to change these lifestyle factors, you can create both health and disease. If you already suffer from a disease, you may wonder if it is too late to salvage your situation. If you don't already have a disease, you may wonder if it is too early to be concerned about it. In either case, ask yourself: First, can the degenerative process be slowed? Second, can the process be halted, so it gets no worse? And third, can the process be reversed, undoing some of the already existing damage?

Accomplishing any one of these is a step toward longevity, an enhanced quality of life, and a decreased need for outside intervention and medications. The good news is that deterioration can usually be slowed, halted, or reversed. The sooner you address lifestyle factors that lead toward optimal function, the better. Your goal is to anticipate your own good health versus reacting to—or even creating—disease.

If you equate good health with the absence of overt symptoms and become concerned about your health only if something hurts or stops working, you're operating under a health-versus-disease mindset. But the absence of overt symptoms is not the same as optimal health. Since we are programmed for survival, our bodies somehow find ways to keep going, which, in itself, convinces us that everything must be just fine. But though our bodies are masterful at adapting to adverse circumstances, the continued adaptations often carry an unrecognized expense.

When you come to see good health as not just the absence of symptoms but a state of optimal function and well-being, you'll start to see your health differently: you'll see degrees of health, based on levels of normal function versus dysfunction. And your relative degree of health translates into your daily performance and productivity, even into how you feel from moment to moment.

You can actually postpone, minimize, and sometimes eliminate the onset of degenerative disease through how you live each day! Yes, you have your genetic blueprint, but what you do with it is what really counts. A healthy lifestyle and a well-maintained, properly functioning body can indeed slow your aging process while delaying the onset and reducing the severity of chronic disease!

The Lifestyle Syndrome

While the United States has the highest per capita expenditures on healthcare, it ranks tenth or lower among the world's other twenty-eight industrialized countries in indicators such as life expectancy and infant mortality.[5] Spending on healthcare has led to less health, and a large part of the growing health problem, which is the increase in and earlier onset of chronic disease—is self-induced. Since this problem is a product of our lifestyles and is reinforced by cultural attitudes and practices, it is not likely to be solved by the existing complex of medical industries, government, and private insurance.

A 2004 report in the *Journal of the American Medical Association* entitled "The Actual Causes of Death in the United States, 2000" investigated modifiable behavioral risk factors. The results: Although smoking remains the leading cause of death, poor diet and physical inactivity are close behind and may soon overtake it.[6]

Often, what we regard as disease is actually a plethora of degenerative conditions that are predictable outcomes of our very own lifestyles. There is even a medical term, *lifestyle syndrome*, that defines the poor habits many of us consider to be normal. It is defined as "a cluster of conditions and diseases that result from consuming too many calories; ingesting too much saturated fat, sodium and alcohol; not expending enough calories (inactivity and lack of exercise); and using tobacco or being exposed to tobacco smoke. In addition to hypertension, manifestations of the lifestyle syndrome include the metabolic syndrome, obesity, dyslipidemia

7

(cholesterol and other fat imbalances), cardiovascular disease, cancer, osteoarthritis, depression, sexual dysfunction, and type 2 diabetes mellitus."[7]

The lifestyle syndrome stems from Western culture's obsession with immediate gratification and instant relief, regardless of long-term effects, and with getting ahead in a world where winning the battle has become more important than winning the war. In addition, principles and practices of health are neither taught nor modeled in our schools; diets that include foods devoid of nutrients and loaded with refined sugar, bad fats, and artificial chemical additives are the norm; and we implicitly teach our children that exercise and physical activity are not important because we have neither the time nor funding for meaningful physical education in schools. All of this has enormous repercussions on your and your loved ones' life spans and tomorrow's medical costs. Many existing attitudes toward health have been shaped by medical and pharmaceutical approaches that evolved during the twentieth century. An historic event occurred in 1964 with the discovery that a chemical called a beta-blocker, which blocked some of the effects of our own adrenaline, could be effective in controlling elevated blood pressure. Since this condition, also known as hypertension, can produce strokes (the third most frequent cause of death in the United States), beta-blockers were deemed a godsend.

The downside of this miracle was that millions of us could artificially reduce our high blood pressure without addressing the cause of our hypertension. Logical questions went unanswered: Why are my adrenal glands producing too much of the hormones that raise blood pressure? And what can be done to normalize the function of my adrenal glands so they no longer produce an excess of blood-pressure-elevating stress hormones?

Forty years later we still don't ask these questions. If you are diagnosed with elevated blood pressure, you will likely routinely take pills to block the effects of a hormone your own body is producing in excess, never thinking to address the lifestyle factors that cause the problem in the first place.

But what if you addressed your high blood pressure by modifying lifestyle factors such as how much water you drink, how much salt

8

and minerals you take in, how much caffeine you consume, your exercise or lack of it, and measures you could take to reduce or off-set your stress levels so that your adrenal glands return to normal levels of hormonal production?

Sure, the pill may sound easier, but at some point, you have to pay the pill-popping piper. Refusing to address and improve crucial lifestyle factors winds up predisposing you to a host of other chronic degenerative disorders. Ironically, the magical beta-blockers and other pills that let us ignore the impact of our poor lifestyles have helped create a ticking time bomb of degenerative disorders that threatens not just your own future health but also the overall levels of health and prosperity in our society today.

Our ability to medicate ourselves has mushroomed into a pervasive use and reliance on pharmaceuticals to control symptoms and treat disorders that arise from the lifestyle syndrome. Can medications to lower cholesterol, for example, be taken long-term without side effects? If you are currently taking such a medication, did you realize that you are a participant in a long-term research study? For many drugs, the results are currently unknown as to their overall effectiveness versus their potential side effects, including interactions with other drugs you may take, as related to your own genetic uniqueness. It might be safer for you to address your lifestyle as well as potential malfunctions in your body that could have caused the elevated levels of cholesterol in the first place.

Don't ignore the principles of good health while assuming that technology will one day discover ways to undo the inevitable damage from an unhealthy lifestyle. The appropriate goal is not to eliminate your need for pharmaceutical intervention but to minimize, delay, and simplify the need for medications.

The Inner Pharmacy

The human body has a phenomenal ability to regulate itself. It constantly produces an array of chemicals that control body functions such as heart rate, blood pressure, blood-sugar and fat levels, digestion, inflammation, expansion of the air passageways for breathing, to name a few of many thousands. Some chemicals are stimulating; others are calming. It is the balance of different chemicals that keep you from feeling overstimulated and anxious, or on the other extreme, fatigued, lethargic, and unmotivated.

Your body maintains an extremely complicated balance of chemicals by controlling the production, utilization, and breakdown of each one. If, for example, you have symptoms related to an excess of a particular chemical, a finite set of possibilities exists to account for that excess. Either your body is producing too much of that chemical or not breaking down enough of that chemical, which often means the body is not utilizing it and not converting it into another chemical that may be necessary to maintain normal function.

When present in excess amounts, a good chemical can act like a bad chemical and, in fact, become one. For instance, chemicals that encourage inflammation and save lives by isolating localized infections can stimulate ongoing inflammation when present in too high amounts for too long. These same pro-inflammatory chemicals are normally balanced by the body's production of anti-inflammatory chemicals. A deficiency in production of anti-inflammatory chemicals can result in too many pro-inflammatory chemicals, making for increased inflammation anywhere in the body. It's all about balance.

Likewise, if you have symptoms of a deficiency of a specific chemical, several possibilities also exist. One is that the gland or tissue responsible for the chemical's production may be malfunctioning. It could be underactive because it is not getting proper stimulation from another area or function of the body. For example, the thyroid gland does not maintain normal levels of function unless stimulated by the pituitary gland. Or a gland could be fatigued from years of overuse, such as a pancreas that has produced a lifetime of insulin by the age of twenty, due to a diet too high in concentrated sugars. Additionally, your body can lose its responsiveness to normal amounts of a chemical after years of exposure to excesses of that chemical. Diets high in concentrated sugars trigger excesses of insulin from the pancreas, which eventually create insulin resistance, where the body is numb or unresponsive to the insulin that is present. The inability of the fatigued pancreas to maintain its normal function or the body's inability to respond to normal amounts of insulin then becomes adult-onset (or type 2) diabetes. It results from an imbalance of the Inner Pharmacy.

A chemical deficiency can also occur from a dearth of the chemical building blocks needed to make it, a common result of a poor-quality diet or a lifestyle that demands more of that chemical than the body can regularly produce. Subsequent chapters will show how a high-adrenaline lifestyle, common to many of us, not only requires more of certain nutrients to sustain itself but also eventually fatigues the adrenal glands from years of overactivity and leads to further chemical deficiencies.

Another key aspect of the body's Inner Pharmacy is that the body produces both good and bad chemicals, although most "bad" chemicals are actually "good" ones that act bad when present in excess amounts. Cholesterol, for example, is not inherently a bad chemical. A normally functioning body uses cholesterol to produce testosterone, estrogen, progesterone, aldosterone, cortisol, and other critical hormones. People think of cholesterol as bad, because its excess contributes to heart disease. But a well-functioning body, supplied with a healthy diet, doesn't have an excess of cholesterol because it uses up both the moderate amounts it is given and the amounts it manufactures on its own in the production of other necessary chemicals. In other words, you have a built-in system of checks and balances that normally sustains your health. But with an unhealthy lifestyle, your body can lose its amazing ability to regulate itself.

In short, your body maintains an intricate balance based on the raw materials you give it and what your Inner Pharmacy manufactures from those ingredients. A malfunction of the body, such as reduced stomach-acid production or an unhealthy lifestyle, can disturb this balance and create a sequence of events that lead to extensive chemical imbalances. These persistent chemical imbalances, if not addressed, can advance, become more complicated, and evolve into what is known as chronic disease. Yes, *almost every chronic disease results, at least in part, from a chemical imbalance within.* When the Inner Pharmacy can no longer maintain balance, the body becomes unable to control itself in a healthy manner.

Options abound for restoring normal function and balance to your body and your lifestyle, thereby allowing your Inner Pharmacy to produce more good chemicals to regulate itself and maintain your health. The other option is the external pharmacy—the store down the street. But even if an imbalance is already advanced and has been regulated with medications for a long time, your health will benefit when you optimize whatever amount of normal function still exists. Let's explore how to maximize your body's normal functions, using a familiar example.

The Attack of the Saber-Toothed Tiger

The fight-or-flight response is often described in basic biology courses to demonstrate how the human body responds to emergencies. The scenario commonly described starts with our human ancestors, millions of years ago, calmly sitting around the cave when suddenly they are attacked by a saber-toothed tiger.

The threat of the tiger stimulates an immediate response in their nervous and hormonal (neuroendocrine) systems. In this instant, they do not ponder various escape routes and consider where they will end up and what they might have for dinner next week. *They simply react.* A rush of adrenaline creates immediate and dramatic shifts throughout their bodies, diverting their energy and function into surviving the urgent, current situation.

Immediate effects include increased heart rate and blood pressure, elevated blood sugar, bronchodilation (expansion of the air passageways), dilation of the pupils, and heightened awareness of the present moment. The body's priorities shift from day-to-day functions such as digestion and energy storage to the mobilization of stored energy to aid survival.

While such survival mechanisms have their time and place, imagine your life if you were attacked by a saber-toothed tiger several times a day, year after year. You would certainly be preoccupied with your current and ongoing issue of survival and not necessarily be thinking clearly about your future. Your nervous system would constantly be activating the survival mechanisms that allow you to either fight or flee from the current attack.

While you may still be alive at the end of each day, your body would be making huge trade-offs because *the very mechanisms engaged by your body for survival in an emergency are the same ones that accelerate the aging process and deplete your reserves for the future*. And the frequent or almost constant activation of these survival mechanisms contributes to the five chronic diseases most responsible for driving up healthcare costs: heart disease, hypertension, diabetes, asthma, and mood disorders. Many other common symptoms, such as heartburn and digestive problems, elevated cholesterol, fatigue, anxiety and depression, arthritis, and inflammatory disorders can also be traced directly to an over-activation of the stress response. The U.S. national Centers for Disease Control estimates that 90 percent of visits to all types of doctors are for stress-related illnesses.[8]

In the twenty-first century, the saber-toothed tiger lives on in many forms that may be eating you alive, not in one big gulp but in small nibbling bites. Your body reacts to the honking horn of the frazzled driver behind you just as your ancestors reacted to the tiger. Whether it is the "hurry up and wait" frustrations of daily commutes, the rushed pace of life in general, or the enormous bombardment of information (mostly bad news), your survival mechanisms react as if a tiger is attacking you. The chemical stresses of nutrient-depleted foods loaded with refined sugars, trans fats, and other chemical additives add to the cumulative effect that your body perceives as an attacking tiger.

Frequent attacks of the saber-toothed tiger not only damage your health, they alter your entire life by distorting your perspective and shifting your priorities. When the tiger attacks, you don't consciously shift your priorities. Instead, your body's preprogrammed responses do that for you, whether you want them to or not. Your neurochemical responses, triggered by the tiger, change your perception of time and limit your ability to logically and sensibly plan for your future. Depending on your stress level and what you have or have not done to offset it, you may not be thinking clearly about what is really important over the span of your life. Being under frequent attacks by the tiger actually limits your choices and decision-making abilities and shortens both the quality and quantity of your life. Instinctive survival behaviors are emphasized at the expense of your humanness.

Figure 2 shows the human body's immediate responses to stress, whether the stress is a saber-toothed tiger or a one-hour commute in stop-and-go traffic.

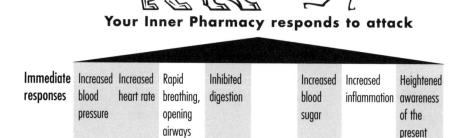

Your Inner Pharmacy responds to attack

Immediate responses	Increased blood pressure	Increased heart rate	Rapid breathing, opening airways	Inhibited digestion		Increased blood sugar	Increased inflammation	Heightened awareness of the present

Figure 2

Each of the involuntary changes in your body as it responds to the tiger is chemically based, a product of your Inner Pharmacy. Some responses to stress don't appear until minutes or hours later; these are shown as "delayed responses" in figure 3.

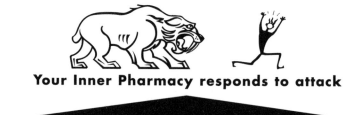

Your Inner Pharmacy responds to attack

Immediate responses	Increased blood pressure	Increased heart rate	Rapid breathing, opening airways	Inhibited digestion		Increased blood sugar	Increased inflammation	Heightened awareness of the present
Delayed responses	Increased blood clotting	Increased blood fats			Enhanced immunity			Anxiety

Figure 3

Next, you can see in figure 4 under "prolonged responses" how prolonged activation of the stress response (the lifestyle syndrome) can create imbalances and damage. Chronic diseases result when the Inner Pharmacy is chronically stimulated to manufacture too many bad chemicals or an excess of certain chemicals. In fact, the top five chronic diseases (high blood pressure, heart disease, asthma, diabetes, and mood disorders) all have a direct link to the frequent activation of the body's stress response. The continued stress erodes the body's ability to regulate itself, and health gradually turns into disease. Which body parts and/or mechanisms break down first determine which chronic disease you develop, as influenced by your genetic weak links. For some people, it is the digestive system; for others, it may be the heart and vascular system, or the joints.

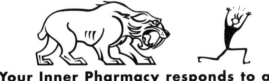

Your Inner Pharmacy responds to attack

Immediate responses	Increased blood pressure	Increased heart rate	Rapid breathing, opening airways	Inhibited digestion		Increased blood sugar	Increased inflammation	Heightened awareness of the present
Delayed responses	Increased blood clotting	Increased blood fats			Enhanced immunity			Anxiety
Prolonged responses	Increased blood pressure, increased plaque in blood vessels, heart disease, cerebrovascular disease, stroke		Asthma, chronic respiratory disease	Heartburn, GERD	Inhibited immunity, chronic illness, flu, fatigue, pneumonia	Diabetes, insulin resistance	Any "itis" condition, arthritis	Anxiety, depression, mood disorders

Figure 4

During prolonged activation of the stress response, some of your body's mechanisms become depleted and eventually produce symptoms which can be the opposite of the initial response. For example, when the Inner Pharmacy can no longer maintain an adrenaline high, depression often results. Or when cortisol, an adrenal stress hormone, continues to be produced in excess, it inhibits or weakens the immune system, making you more vulnerable to illness. Or asthma, the constriction of air passageways, can result when the body can no longer maintain stress-induced bronchodilation, or expansion of air passageways.

The fact that day-to-day life in technologically advanced countries is producing so much chronic disease is a system failure. How we live our lives, including some deeply ingrained cultural attitudes, may be seriously compromising our health and well-being. It raises obvious questions, one of which is, where do we go from here?

But before we address that question, let's look at an even greater system failure: how Western medicine deals with chronic disease. Western medicine tries to solve the new epidemic of chronic disease with an old solution developed in the twentieth century for acute and infectious disease. As shown in figure 5, the old-paradigm approach of "treating the disease" means that medications are given to treat or control the prolonged responses listed in the diagram, in other words, the symptoms of chronic illness. But remember, these symptoms and the illness itself are primarily being created by an imbalance of the Inner Pharmacy, a result of its having been overstimulated by too many tigers too frequently. Medications rarely address the causes of the imbalance.

Of course, treating the disease is a valid approach once the body can no longer regulate itself, and it plays a vital role in managing chronic disease. Yet, when chronic disease is our number-one health problem, and much of it is due to the self-inflicted lifestyle syndrome, it is time for a new approach to health, one that doesn't merely manage but prevents.

The New Paradigm: Taming the Saber-Toothed Tiger

A more holistic approach to chronic disease is simple: to treat the person who has the disease instead of treating the disease. Much

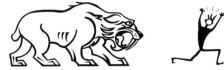

Your Inner Pharmacy responds to attack

Immediate responses	Increased blood pressure	Increased heart rate	Rapid breathing, opening airways	Inhibited digestion		Increased blood sugar	Increased inflammation	Heightened awareness of the present
Delayed responses	Increased blood clotting	Increased blood fats			Enhanced immunity			Anxiety
Prolonged responses	Increased blood pressure, increased plaque in blood vessels, heart disease, cerebrovascular disease, stroke		Asthma, chronic respiratory disease	Heartburn, GERD	Inhibited immunity, chronic illness, flu, fatigue, pneumonia	Diabetes, insulin resistance	Any "itis" condition, arthritis	Anxiety, depression, mood disorders

Medications
The old paradigm is to use medications to treat the symptoms of chronic disease.

Figure 5

more than a matter of semantics, treating the person is quite different from treating the disease. Treating the person means working to shift your Inner Pharmacy to produce a different set of chemicals, which then produce a different set of effects. These chemicals, produced by your own Inner Pharmacy, lead to normal function, as the body controls and maintains its own healthy blood pressure, heart rate, breathing, digestion, immune function, blood sugar, inflammation, and moods. Treating the person rather than the disease has tremendous potential to improve your health as well as to help you avoid and prevent disease. This may be obvious, but it is the essence of longevity, endurance, and healthy aging.

For yourself, what does it mean to treat the person? It means sharing responsibility for your health with your physician. You, not just your doctor, take an active role in creating and maintaining your own health. (Parts 2 and 3 provide a guide to options and actions to help you.) Treating the person has three essential components:

1. *Raw materials.* A good diet (including dietary supplements such as vitamins) provides your Inner Pharmacy with the materials it needs to produce good chemicals and rebuild damaged and fatigued organs. A good diet also eliminates food sensitivities.

2. *A healthy lifestyle.* This includes exercise, especially aerobic exercise, to convert good fats into energy and anti-inflammatory chemicals. A healthy lifestyle also includes recreation and other means of stress reduction such as yoga to reduce the effects of the tigers in your life. It includes artistic pursuits to stimulate both sides of your brain. Your lifestyle—how you use your body— determines what your Inner Pharmacy does with the raw materials you give it.

3. *Healthcare and body maintenance.* Your goal is to maintain the normal function of your body. The healthcare you choose also determines what your Inner Pharmacy can do with the raw materials you provide it. This means using healthcare that works to restore and maintain normal function, such as

   - Chiropractic treatment and a wellness program to correct misalignments and malfunctions and to maintain the health of your spine and nervous system
   - Applied Kinesiology to correct the function of your feet, knees, pelvis, and diaphragm (which increases oxygen to the brain and tissues) and to rebuild damaged or fatigued organs
   - Craniosacral treatment to stimulate the parasympathetic nervous system
   - Acupuncture to promote harmony and balance of your electromagnetic energy

- Neuro Emotional Technique to realign your emotional congruence with health and healthy goals
- Naturopathy and homeopathy
- Massage and other bodywork

The tiger has not been magically eliminated. Stress is universal and eternal. But an important concept is that stress is not all bad. A small to moderate amount is stimulating, invigorating, productive, and healthy. Hans Selye, the original researcher and pioneer in the field of stress, distinguished between good stress, which he termed *eustress*, and excess stress that produces damage, or *distress*. Examples of eustress are a goal or a deadline that forces you to focus on a project. A healthy body and attitude can thrive indefinitely on eustress. However, years of distress can wear down the healthiest of bodies and dampen the strongest of spirits.

Your goal is not to eliminate the tiger but to tame it to reduce its damaging effects. You can tame the tiger by strengthening and fortifying yourself so you are less vulnerable to the tigers that are out there. Some of the elements described above, such as yoga, artistic pursuits, or massage, fortify you. A calm, centered, and healthy person is much less affected by the same stress that would upset someone who is in pain, frazzled, and eating improperly.

Your goal is also to reduce the number of tigers in your life and the frequency of their attacks. Your body responds to excess carbohydrates, caffeine, alcohol, trans fats, and other poor diet choices as if each is one more tiger. Therefore, a good and balanced diet reduces the number of tigers your Inner Pharmacy needs to respond to.

As shown in items 2 and 3 above, you naturally offset existing stress through play, exercise, and by choosing a combination of Western medicine and complementary or alternative medicine (CAM) to promote the normal, balanced function of your body.

This new healthy approach to health is about *you*, not your *disease*. You are your Inner Pharmacy. Shifting your Inner Pharmacy to produce fewer bad chemicals and more good chemicals has enormous benefits. It means not only that you are likely to reduce your current annoying symptoms but also that you are taking appropriate steps to reduce other symptoms and to delay the onset of any chronic diseases as well.

This bonus from treating the person is distinctly different from what happens when you treat a disease. Treating the person is the essence of prevention and wellness. Complementary and alternative medicine is philosophically congruent with health and wholeness; its growing acceptance—most insurance companies now pay for these services—is due not only to its effectiveness in treating people's physical ailments but also because it often helps them in secondary ways they did not anticipate. For instance, treating a person for a stomach problem frequently improves joint problems as well. It also commonly helps with fatigue, because the same imbalance in the body may be producing the stomach problem, the fatigue, and some of the joint problems.

While some chronic diseases such as osteoarthritis are considered to be a normal part of the aging process, improving your health can delay or postpone their onset and even minimize their severity, especially in light of the fact that many adult-onset diseases such as diabetes are now widely occurring at earlier ages, even in children.

A more holistic approach to health doesn't mean abandoning traditional Western medicine. Rather, it uses it as part of a larger health system that treats the person, not just the disease, in order to improve overall health. Treating the person who has the disease means controlling their symptoms and keeping them safe and healthy. If the body has deteriorated to a point where it can no longer control itself, of course medications are indicated as necessary.

If you are already taking medications to manage a chronic disease, complement this traditional approach by treating your whole self, not just your symptoms. If, on the other hand, you are reasonably healthy and not already suffering from a chronic disease, it is wise to seek healthcare that treats your whole person, not any symptoms you may have, and to use traditional Western medical approaches if more extreme intervention becomes necessary.

If you are a cancer survivor, you are very likely alive today because of early detection of the disease and sophisticated medications and treatments. Though the lifestyle syndrome triggers many cancers, any major acute disease or injury has a way of catching our attention and refocusing us on our health priorities. If you have vanquished cancer, you can aggressively re-create your health using the more holistic approach described in this book, one that focuses on the health of your whole being.

A big difference exists between doing nothing about your health and doing something. Many people do nothing because they don't know what to do. Still others know a few things and do nothing because they lack discipline or commitment. Let's proceed to improve your health, not because it's what you should do but because it's the only realistic option for creating a life and quality time to enjoy it.

2

UNDERSTANDING HEALTH

Creating health isn't much more difficult than creating disease. From the moment you were born, you have been creating both, in varying degrees. So creating health isn't some new and foreign project to take on. It is a matter of accentuating certain natural health-promoting activities and discontinuing others that are destructive and disease-promoting. It is a matter of asking the right questions, of restoring and maintaining a well-functioning body, and of living your daily life in a way that nurtures and sustains your physical health and your mental well-being.

Creating Health and Disease

You are creating health and disease right now. At this very moment, you are expressing your own genetic uniqueness through the way you are living. At this moment your own Inner Pharmacy is producing good and not-so-good chemicals, based on the genes you inherited and on what you are doing to amplify protective genes and inactivate those that predispose you to disease. "What you are doing" includes what you've been eating (and for that matter, when you ate it), because what you ingest constitutes the raw materials your body has available to make hormones, enzymes, neurotransmitters, and even chemicals that reduce inflammation. "What you are doing" also includes the spectrum of your physical, mental, and emotional activities. When and how you exercised last, for instance, has a distinct bearing on what chemicals your body is producing and what ratio of fat and sugars you are burning at this moment to sustain and propel your life.

All this determines not just the quality of your current experience but the cumulative wear and tear on your body. For most of us, it's this largely self-induced wearing out of parts that contributes to degeneration, aging, and the premature decline of body function. What we eat, how we move, how we think and feel, and how we train our bodies to produce more of certain chemicals and less of others all makes a difference in the quality and productivity of our present lives and the likelihood that we'll be able to enjoy our future—*or even have one!* The way in which we deal, or don't deal, with the inevitable stressors in our life not only directly influences neurotransmitter levels (and our corresponding emotional moods and states of awareness) but literally impacts the level of inflammation we're experiencing throughout our bodies. Yes, at this very moment you are actively forging your health destiny.

Ironically, the ongoing process of crafting your own health destiny, if you're like most people, is the furthest thing from your mind. But it is perhaps the most important life work you can conduct. Unfortunately, most of us generally focus on our health only when we suddenly fear it's failing or when we're prompted by a specific symptom—a lump in the breast, or a stiff knee. When a complaint manifests itself, we may sweat out whether it means something ominous and whether we should be doing something about it rather than vainly trying to ignore it. If it frightens us sufficiently, we may even have it investigated. It's typically only during these anxious times that we consider being on good health behavior for a while, such as improving our diet or level of exercise or perhaps eliminating some bad habit. If the symptom is found to be insignificant or if it simply disappears, we typically breathe a sigh of relief and comfortably return to our existing habits and lifestyle. It is a tragedy that without the drama of life-threatening disease hanging over us, plans to improve our health are typically short-lived.

Most of us have never been trained to look at health. We don't learn much about it in school or in the workplace. Unfortunately, many of us have been forced to look squarely at disease far more often than we have looked at health. Whether it's yourself or a loved one, the threat of disease reliably seizes your attention and focuses you on the value of health. People too often wake up to the value of their health when it is too late to save a life. If health is salvageable, a much better quality of life could often have been preserved with less work and expense if that individual had made health a greater priority earlier on.

None of us was born with a government-issued warranty to cover the parts of our body for a hundred years or an instruction manual for periodic maintenance. And it is because of the lack of proper maintenance that many parts of the body become dysfunctional or wear out prematurely. When they do, they require either replacement or a pharmaceutical prescription. We, as a culture, have abdicated our responsibility for our own health with the now-common idea that it is the responsibility of the government, private insurance, and the medical system to provide these solutions, regardless of our own failure to care for and maintain our health throughout life.

A more enlightened approach is to take responsibility for your own health by establishing a healthy lifestyle and working to promote optimal function of all body parts. It's odd that many people seem to understand the concept of optimal function in the realm of consumer items, such as cars, kitchen appliances, computers, or sound systems, but it's not a concept applied to our own bodies.

Throughout our time on earth, our greatest resource is our health. It gives us the opportunity to experience and enjoy life, to love and be loved. Future security does not come just from money in the bank. It requires feeling good, physically and mentally. No amount of money can buy the security that derives from enduring good health.

Time is the one thing that money can't buy. When we're young, time seems limitless, but at some point, time moves to the top of our list of most valued "possessions." We all want more of it. But if money can't buy time, how can you obtain more of it? Simple: One definition of the word *buy* is "to obtain in exchange for something." The exchange that buys time is attention to your health, a healthy lifestyle, and use of healthcare resources to optimize the function of all parts of your body for as long as possible. Time and health can be earned, invested, and experienced later.

As babies and then young children, we come into this world and we play. We are naturally physically active as we explore the world. We are inherently driven to move, to crawl, to walk on our own. And to run! Yet at some point, we begin moving less and less. Some would say we stop moving because we get older. The truth is we get older faster because we stop moving and exploring. One big factor in the lifestyle syndrome is a scarcity of stress-reducing activities (i.e., fun!) to offset the stresses of modern life. Healthy aging is a way of life that requires recreation, fun, and play.

Healthy aging does not require you to craft a perfect lifestyle. A vibrant 99-year-old gentleman was asked the secret to his longevity. He replied, "Moderation in all things—with a few marvelous exceptions." What you do six days a week is more important than what you do once a week. The cumulative effects of your regular health-promoting activities will help to neutralize or cancel the ill effects of many disease-producing activities.

If you save money for retirement, you expect that your savings will provide financial support to enjoy the golden years. In an informal survey of my patients, affluent, older individuals who had sufficient savings were asked what they valued most. The answer, almost universally, was "quality time with family and loved ones in a beautiful, natural environment." Perhaps, then, even more important than regular financial contributions to a retirement account are daily contributions of attention, time, and energy to your "healthy aging" fund. Let's look next at the how your contributions to a healthy aging fund can actually create quality time.

Buy Time through Healthy Aging

Consider how productive you could be in the course of each day if you had a steady supply of energy, no pain or discomfort to distract you, and the ability to focus for long periods on tasks at hand. This is quality time—time not unlike the state of life you enjoyed as a child, when your energy was endless and your health unencumbered. When your metabolism and nervous system are functioning effectively, you can achieve this maximized state for many years beyond what most of us have come to expect. You are creating quality time.

You can postpone age-related disability by reducing your lifestyle risk factors and implementing health-promoting activities. A recent study compared two groups of adults at an average age of 68 years. One group exercised, had normal body-mass indexes, and did not smoke. The other group did not exercise, was obese, and smoked tobacco. The healthier lifestyle group postponed disability by 7.75 years over the other group.[1] It is likely that the greatest declines in disability in the coming decades will result more from reductions in lifestyle risk factors than any sudden miraculous medical breakthroughs. Add to this the fact that the cost of your medical care if you become a disabled older person will average three times the cost for a non-disabled senior, and it becomes apparent that all of us have a vested interest in working toward a healthy lifestyle.[2]

As early as 1948, visionary medical doctor and researcher Jeremiah Stamler witnessed the effects of risk factors in laboratory animals and made the connection between diet and cardiovascular disease.[3] Since heart disease, a leading killer of both men and women, is an ongoing, degenerative process in which genetic risk factors are activated by lifestyle triggers and accentuated by increased inflammation, it's critical to address the variables that can modify our bodies' degenerative processes through diet, lifestyle, and proper function of our bodies. That is the essence of healthy aging; it may be the only way to buy or create time.

Postponing the decline in body function allows you to maintain a high quality of life beyond the normal biological limits of old age. No longer just a theory, the possibility of adding quality years to your life is now a well-documented phenomenon.[4] In 1980, James Fries, M.D., of the Stanford University School of Medicine, used the phrase, "squaring the survival curve," meaning that instead of spending the second half of your life in gradually declining health, your goal is to postpone disability and live a higher quality of life for a longer period of time.[5] The end of life may come more abruptly when some vital function fails, but it comes after more good years of healthy living.

"We live too short and die too long" describes the current approach to aging. You can turn this on its head and "live longer and die shorter." Rather than spending the second half of your life in a gradual decline, or perhaps the last decades of life seriously disabled, you can optimize your genetic gifts and opportunities through how you live. Here are three strategies for healthy aging.

Three steps to buy time

There are three steps you can take to buy more time. First, begin asking the right questions. When you have a pain or symptom, rather than ask, "What medication do I need to take?" inquire beyond the obvious and ask yourself a few questions such as "What is malfunctioning in my body to create the symptom?" "What isn't working properly in my body or my lifestyle to create this problem?" and "Is it fixable? Can it be corrected by some treatment or lifestyle modification?" Try this for heartburn, joint pain, elevated blood pressure, high cholesterol, fatigue, anxiety, or depression.

This approach does not mean you should ignore any symptom or attempt to become your own doctor. It just means that you ask logical and fundamental questions of yourself and your doctors. It means you take responsibility for being part of the cause as well as the solution. "Do it for me; give me a pill to make my problem go away" doesn't work for chronic disease. What will work is normalizing the function of your Inner Pharmacy through healthy living and health-promoting maintenance of your body. For most chronic disease and non-life-threatening symptoms, opportunities exist to improve health and create quality time. So start by asking the right questions. For example, many joint pains are due to a mechanical misalignment of the joint or failure of surrounding muscles to support the joint or an acid-base imbalance causing excess calcium to deposit. Any of these are correctible. If you know what to ask, you can be part of the solution to normalize your body's functioning.

The second way to buy time is care and maintenance of your body. If you are like most people, you probably have more routine maintenance performed on your car than you do on your body. Yet your body is subject to wear and tear, just like your car. For example, the body has "shock absorbers" in the feet and ankles. When working properly, nerve endings, called mechanoreceptors, in the feet and ankles contribute to balance, coordination, and normal muscle function throughout the body. When your car has been in an accident, a realignment of the suspension and wheels is often needed. Without realignment, the car runs poorly and less efficiently. Parts (such as the tires) wear out faster than they should. Likewise, in the human body, common sprains and strains that are not treated properly and do not fully heal lead to a lifetime of poor shock absorption that creates premature degeneration of knees, hips, and spine. Improper alignment of vertebrae in the spine and other joints in the body due to falls, injuries, accidents, traumas, and poor posture creates excessive wear and tear on the mechanics of the body and leads to deteriorating function of the nervous system and its control of all body parts. Healthy aging is keeping all parts of your body working as well as possible for as long as possible, and routine maintenance for your body is a way to accomplish that. Many holistic healthcare professionals such as chiropractors and osteopaths do specific corrections on the body to help restore normal function, even after years of neglect. We'll discuss more specifics in parts 2 and 3.

It's important to proactively seek healthcare after injuries because unhealed sprains and strains define the aging process. Besides the increased wear and tear and early deterioration of joints, due to poor shock absorption and misalignments, many of us just give up on exercise because it becomes a miserable experience that feels like we are doing more harm than good. Unfortunately, once we give up on exercise and activity, the aging process accelerates. Do you want that to happen at forty? Or one hundred? One of exercise's greatest benefits is increased oxygenation of the entire body by the action of the diaphragm muscle. If you want your brain to stay sharp, see that it gets more oxygen on a regular basis from daily exercise and a properly functioning body, including the diaphragm muscle. To make exercise a pleasure, keep your body functioning at its optimum by regular healthcare that promotes health instead of just addressing disease.

The third way to buy time is a healthy lifestyle, including diet and nutritional supplements (raw materials for your Inner Pharmacy) as well as exercise, recreation, and stress reduction (which determine what your Inner Pharmacy does with those raw materials). Creating a healthy lifestyle does not require a radical change in how you live. It can easily be done by making your health a priority. It is reframing health and what health means to you in the bigger picture of your whole life. Health takes on a new meaning when you realize that it is the only way to create time.

Health planning: Investing in your future years

There's a parallel between your personal finances and personal health. Spending more than you make and loading up on loans and credit-card debt sacrifices future financial ease for immediate gratification, a situation not so different from sacrificing tomorrow's health for whatever seemingly urgent situation exists today. Debt and savings—here's how they look when it comes to your health.

Lessen your health debt with a sound health plan. A health debt arises when you have compromised longevity and future quality of life for some immediate gain. Ignoring your health, while treating only symptoms of chronic disease, increases your health debt. Retiring your health debt means living in a way that optimizes your genetic potential, not compromises it.

A common-sense approach to save money for the future is to save 10 percent of your income. But how to save 10 percent when there are bills, recreation, and emergencies? Simple, the experts say: *Pay yourself first.* Set up a savings plan in which 10 percent is automatically routed to your account or else have the discipline to set aside the 10 percent before you pay the monthly bills. The same applies to your health. If you wait until the end of the day to see if you have time left to exercise, it is unlikely to happen. If you wait until next week, next month, or next year to improve your diet or initiate a stress-reduction program, that day may never come.

Here is a simple lesson in attitude from a health-conscious friend. When praised for his discipline in maintaining a daily exercise regimen, he replies that missing a day of exercise is not even an option.

Like brushing his teeth, it isn't something he mentally decides to do each day, but rather it's a mental shift born of his awareness of his own body and the priority he gives to his own health and vitality. Perhaps his decision was made easier because he hates how he feels when he doesn't exercise and loves how he feels when he does. Missing a day of exercise is not even a choice in his mind. To improve your health and increase your chances of a secure future, there really isn't a choice.

Creating a healthy lifestyle—health planning—is the theme of part 3. Investing just 10 percent of your leisure time—about five hours a week for most of us—into health-promoting activities is like putting routine deposits into a time bank. Your investment in yourself accumulates and earns compound interest. Dividends come almost immediately in the form of greater energy, clarity, and productivity. As years pass, you get the return on your investment: more good years of health, vitality, and quality of life.

Part 2

Healthcare for Life

3

AN INTEGRATED SYSTEM OF HEALTHCARE

The field of medicine works to prevent and to treat disease. It differs from true *healthcare*, which promotes health and optimal function of the body. In this book I make a distinction between traditional Western medicine (TWM) and complementary and alternative medicine (CAM). TWM is what medicine has looked like, for most of us in Western nations, over the past century. CAM, by definition, complements TWM and includes such approaches to health as acupuncture, homeopathy, and craniosacral therapy, and treatments that vary from Chinese herbalism, a practice which dates back thousands of years, to chiropractic, a newer treatment modality that many now consider mainstream and which dates from 1895. Once considered to be irrelevant, the worth of these approaches has been validated by none other than most major medical insurance companies, which now provide coverage for alternative healthcare.

In both TWM and CAM, diagnostic thought processes are similar, but treatments are usually quite different. TWM is primarily symptom-based: a physician's investigation is predicated on finding the source of a symptom. This investigation can be a simple office visit or an elaborate battery of high-technology tests. If the cause of the symptom is not life-threatening or indicative of a serious disease process, as is the case with chronic diseases such as headaches, joint pain, or heartburn, the symptom itself is usually treated with medication. If the cause is not considered significant enough to warrant medication or surgery, patients are often told that no treatment is available. Yet the degenerative process of chronic disease continues, and pain and discomfort often persist. The limitation of this traditional approach is the black-and-white view of "health versus disease," ignoring the whole gray zone of dysfunction that precedes disease, as we saw in the health continuum in figure 1 on page 5.

CAM professions, such as chiropractic and acupuncture, are generally more dysfunction-based: the investigative process asks first what is malfunctioning in the body to produce this symptom, and second, what can be done to restore normal function so the body can correct or control this symptom on its own. The CAM practitioner seeks to correct the dysfunction, restore normal function, and perhaps support that function in the future with nutritional supplements or exercise/therapy. The chiropractor or manipulative osteopath treats by correcting dysfunctions of a biomechanical nature in the cranium, spine, pelvis, and other joints. The acupuncturist or doctor of Oriental medicine treats by correcting dysfunctions or imbalances in the electromagnetic energy flowing through the body's meridians. The nutritionist, herbalist, or bodyworker treats by correcting dietary imbalances and/or by improving function through specific exercises.

When it comes to diagnostic procedures, technology provides traditional Western medicine with ever-more-sophisticated tools. Treatment procedures, however, are another story. They focus predominantly on sustaining life of the critically ill or injured and on replacing diseased or "worn-out" parts. At this, TWM's treatments are most effective. But for the chronically ill, a CAM approach often has more to offer to aid the restoration of normal function in the body.

The best scenario for healthcare embodies a combination of TWM and CAM. The term "Integrative Medicine" (IM) is often used to describe this. Another commonly used term, "Functional Medicine" (FM), conveys an approach to health and disease that focuses on whatever abnormal function may exist. CAM applies if the interpretation is something that is "complementary to" or "alternative to" medicine. Regardless of the name ultimately settled upon, this evolving field will pursue a functional thought process that seeks to identify or correct a new or chronic symptom.

As the person ultimately responsible for your own health, you can follow a functional thought process and ask questions such those following when you seek help from a healthcare provider:

1. What is causing my problem?
2. Is something in my body not working properly?
3. Is it due to something I am doing—or not doing?
4. What can I and my healthcare provider do to correct it?
5. If medication is suggested,
   a. Will the medication correct the problem?
   b. How long will I need to take it?
   c. Will the medication compromise any other functions in my body or have any side effects?
   d. Will my body work better once I am done with the medication?

If the cause of the symptom is determined to be a malfunction and if greater levels of normal function can be restored, one goal will be to postpone the prolonged use of new medications. This is a different scenario than an already existing severe deterioration, in which medication is necessary to maintain vital function.

Increasingly, people in technologically advanced societies have embraced CAM. A landmark paper published in the *Journal of the American Medical Association* in 1998 showed that in the United States there were more patient visits during 1997 to CAM practitioners (639 million) than visits to TWM providers (489 million).[1] Even amidst this astounding growth in the public's use of CAM services, CAM is still only understood in fragments, and the divergent philosophies and perspectives of TWM and CAM continue to pose the greatest barrier to the creation of a truly integrated system of healthcare. The rest of part 2 will help you to understand the philosophy underlying CAM's more holistic approach to healthcare.

4

THE MISSING PIECE IN YOUR HEALTHCARE

Your Inner Pharmacy's production of good chemicals depends on three critical factors: raw materials, your lifestyle (both the subject of part 3), and the normal function of your body. Normal function means that the body controls and maintains, on its own, vital functions such as blood pressure, heart rate, breathing, digestion, immune function, blood sugar, inflammation, and moods. When your Inner Pharmacy is unable to regulate these functions, as in the case of hypertension (elevated blood pressure), for example, the external pharmacy—drugs—are called upon. Many of us consider it to be normal to take drugs to control chronic symptoms. This is not normal! The goal of this book is to show you how to optimize your health by restoring and maintaining the normal function of your body.

Your body is probably not functioning at 100 percent capacity, or in an optimal way every moment. Optimum function is not merely a matter of health versus disease. ("If I'm not sick, then I must be healthy.") Rather, optimum function of the body is a matter of degrees. We could be operating at just 10 percent of our capacity and without overt symptoms, but is this health? Most of us are not aware of the extent our bodies have been compromised by past injuries and stresses such as sprains, strains, falls, or whiplashes. The road to malfunction of the body and the development of chronic disease is paved, not only by your genes, but by your past traumas, injuries, stresses, and lifestyle imbalances.

The empowering fact is that much of normal function can be returned to your body by correcting the causes of the specific dysfunctions you have acquired. Even years after an injury or the development of an imbalance in the body, corrective procedures can often restore normal function and lessen the damage, thus decreasing the age-related decline that had been accelerated by that imbalance. This is healthcare, and it means caring for health. In this section, we'll look at several examples of real patient encounters.

I'll begin by saying that I look at health. Most patients come to see me to get rid of a pain, digestive problem, fatigue, or another annoying symptom. To help eliminate the person's symptoms, I have to identify what isn't working properly in his or her body or lifestyle. It requires a frame of reference of normal, healthy function and comparing the patient to this template to find out what isn't functioning properly. For example, knowing how spinal supporting muscles work during sitting and standing is a key to revealing abnormal function.

Once the malfunction is identified, I try to correct it or perhaps direct the patient to some lifestyle alterations to fix the problem. Since I don't use medications or surgery, the only way I can help get people better is to find and fix the cause of the problem. Medicine has made great progress in the replacement of body parts, whether it be heart or knees or kidneys. But just as you perform maintenance on your car to extend the life of its parts, my focus is not to replace parts but to keep all the parts of the body working as well as possible for as long as possible. That means looking more at the function of the parts themselves as well as how they work with and communicate with each other.

One area in which CAM and TWM differ is in the goal of diagnosis. TWM focuses on putting a name on a disease process or set of symptoms. In holistic healthcare, it's more important to identify the malfunction causing the symptoms. Following are the two approaches to a common symptom.

A woman comes to the office complaining of frequent and debilitating headaches. The doctor or healthcare provider begins with a case history and examines her to make sure that it isn't a tumor or a disease process that is causing the headaches. Both a CAM and a TWM practitioner might order blood tests or other diagnostic testing or refer the patient if anything seems suspicious. If it seems clear that no dangerous disease is causing the headaches, the approaches then begin to differ.

The TWM approach to headache would likely be to prescribe pain medication and possibly refer the patient to a headache special- ist who may use additional medications or pain-management tech- niques. If the headaches are not too severe, the patient may be encouraged to live with them and to use over-the-counter pain medi- cation as needed.

The CAM approach is quite different. People often ask me, as a CAM provider, if I treat headaches. I usually answer, "No, I don't treat headaches; I treat people who have headaches." I treat the *person* who has the problem. In doing so, I am often able to help people not just with their headaches or primary complaint but with other symptoms as well.

For our hypothetical headache sufferer, I begin with a thorough health history. While a trend in medicine is to dehumanize the doctor- patient relationship, I find enormous value in the time spent listening to and interacting with the patient. I have to consider the dangerous possibilities of cancer or tumor, for example, but since most patients who see me for headaches have already undergone diagnostic testing to rule these out, I focus on what malfunctions could be causing the headaches. I have to constantly think "outside the box" to consider the realm of all possibilities. Then I narrow the list of potential causes through a process of elimination. Later on, I'll explain how I can get very specific information from the patient's body regarding what the problem is and how to correct it. Even though it may sound psychic or intuitive, this is simply using functional neurology—the patient's body as a laboratory itself—to assess what is not working in the patient's body.

Both approaches obtain data about the patient, but it is different data because we ask different questions and measure different things.

Ultimately, success at eliminating the headaches results from "matching the treatment to the patient." One weakness of our healthcare system is the lack of generalists who look at you, the patient, as a whole person. Most of us don't have a generalist healthcare provider, someone who can determine the cause of our problem and then treat it or refer us to the appropriate specialist who treats that problem.

Too many of us with chronic problems wander from one specialist to another based on personal recommendations because a friend or relative may have gotten relief in their headaches from that particular specialist or method.

The limitation here is that the friend's or relative's headaches may have been caused by something very different. If your aunt's headaches are caused by toxicity from a poor diet, she will likely get relief from seeing a good nutritionist who cleans up her diet.

For your boss, whose headaches result from biomechanical problems in his neck, such as misaligned vertebrae and muscle tension, the most successful outcome will come through the treatment of a chiropractor or osteopath who corrects the biomechanics. Your boss probably would not get rid of his headaches by seeing the nutritionist, nor would your aunt, with her toxic headaches, find relief by seeing a chiropractor unless the chiropractor also deals with diet and supplements.

For your sister, whose headaches are caused by an imbalance of her energy, a successful outcome might come through acupuncture treatment.

But how does your sister know to see an acupuncturist, your boss a chiropractor, and your aunt a nutritionist? Very little guidance currently exists to optimize this crucial matching process. The solution to this problem is in a system with more generalists, more diagnosticians, but meanwhile there are few CAM generalists, and TWM continues its trend toward increased specialization.[1]

In the symptom-based TWM approach, ten patients with headaches would all receive similar prescriptions. For those same ten patients, however, a CAM provider such as a chiropractor would be doing ten totally different treatments, each one depending on what was causing the headaches for each person. It isn't realistic to think that everyone with chronic headaches has them due to a deficiency of pain medication. Yet treating the symptom and ignoring the dysfunction assumes just that. The CAM provider has to think in terms of the whole person and their habits and lifestyle in order to eliminate headaches and other chronic problems without using drugs or surgery. With TWM and even some symptom-based CAM approaches, it is far too common to use the "one size fits all" approach to headaches and other chronic conditions without considering many potential causes.

Following are examples of how holistic healthcare can shed light on a number of common chronic problems such as headaches, fatigue, gastroesophageal reflux disease, back pain, foot pain, and shoulder pain by identifying and correcting the malfunction that underlies the symptom.

Mechanical Corrections for Mechanical Injuries

How a sixteen-year-old's debilitating headaches were eliminated by understanding a sports injury

Chris came to my office with headaches so severe he was taking several medications to control the pain. He had dropped out of high school because he was depressed and couldn't function well on the medications. Extensive medical testing, including a CAT scan, indicated that all was essentially normal.

In looking for the cause of the problem, I asked questions I ask for almost any chronic problem, for example, "Do the headaches tend to worsen or lessen at a certain time of day?" If so, this might indicate a blood-sugar relationship or possibly an imbalance of the acupuncture energy, known as chi.

Chris's headaches were pretty constant, but as I took his history, a red flag was raised by his answers. I asked about any recent trauma or injury to his head and neck. I also ask about recent dental procedures and orthodontia in patients with headaches. Certain dental procedures, even those performed correctly, can distort and even misalign bones in the head and neck, which can lead to later problems. I ask patients to let me know when they have extensive dental work so that I can correct or reset misalignments and muscle or energy imbalances that may have been thrown off. Holistic-thinking dentists, recognizing that the mouth affects the whole body, often recommend cranial treatment following dental procedures.

About a year earlier, Chris said he had been playing soccer on a wet day and had "headed" the wet and extra-heavy soccer ball. His headaches began almost immediately. Instead of abating in a few days, they worsened and were still fairly steady a year later. As a holistic practitioner, the source of the headaches was straightforward to me: They had been brought on by physical trauma to Chris's head and neck. Other doctors who Chris had consulted recommended medication. Even though the severity could be moderated by medications, the headaches, in my opinion, were not due to a chemical imbalance; clearly, they had arisen from a mechanical injury. Since they had not subsided in the year since the injury, it seemed likely that the mechanical trauma could have created misalignments of the head and neck.

When I examined Chris, I did in fact find misalignments in the vertebrae in his upper neck and even in his cranial bones. After the first treatment to realign those bones, Chris's headaches began to ease up for the first time since the injury. The corrections to the bones and muscles improved blood circulation to his brain and reduced irritation to the nerves. Over the next few months, a series of treatments further realigned these bones and reset injured muscles. Chris's headaches steadily decreased, and he was able to gradually eliminate the medications. Besides getting over the headaches, his concentration and ability to focus returned, his depression left, and he was able to return to school.

After a year of being severely dysfunctional and unsure if he would ever get better, Chris returned to a normal and healthy life. He had suffered a mechanical injury; the logical solution was a mechanical correction to undo the distortion caused by the injury. It makes perfect sense, yet TWM did not look for the cause of the dysfunction and instead merely tried to medicate the symptoms.

If the wheels on your car were misaligned, causing your tires to wear unevenly, you would get the alignment fixed. Not only is it costly to replace tires, but the car doesn't steer as well when the wheels are misaligned. It could even be dangerous. Yet most of us, when we sprain an ankle or strain our knee, back, or neck, proceed through life not knowing we could probably decrease the "wear and tear" on our bodies and avoid a lot of problems by having our "parts" realigned periodically.

This isn't complicated. It's just different; most people have never heard that cranial bones can become misaligned from an injury. Yet cranial bone manipulation has been performed since the early 1900s, when it was developed by an osteopathic physician. Doctors of chiropractic have been doing adjustments to the upper neck and influencing the cranial bones since 1895. Several different approaches to cranial manipulation have evolved over the past century, and cranial treatment is now performed by chiropractors, osteopaths, and other practitioners. Motion of the skull bones has been measured precisely and is a well-documented fact.[2] Yet it will probably be some time before it is recognized by mainstream medicine.

Cranial bone motion is essential to life and the function of the nervous system. If the cranial bones, which normally move as we breathe in and out, become locked up and don't move properly due to trauma to the skull, you can experience pain, especially in the head, neck, jaw, and shoulders. Even more commonly, cranial dysfunction can produce a variety of symptoms such as poor concentration that arises from compromised blood circulation to the brain, or digestive problems such as bloating or heartburn after a meal.

Cranial bone dysfunction directly affects a portion of the autonomic nervous system called the parasympathetic, which controls day-to-day functions like heart rate, production of digestive enzymes, and even peristalsis in the intestines (the natural, rhythmic movement of the intestines). Essential body functions, such as digestion, are controlled by harmony within the nervous system. A head or spine injury, by affecting the nervous system, can interfere with digestion. In the intestines, the sympathetic nerves of the autonomic nervous system inhibit peristalsis, and the parasympathetic nerves stimulate it. An imbalance between the two systems, in which one is overactive and the other underactive, could result in either diarrhea or constipation or even colitis.

Here's another example of how disharmony in the nervous system can affect normal functions such as the stomach's production of acid. There has been an enormous increase in the incidence of heartburn and gastric reflux over the past thirty years—thanks to daily assaults by our modern saber-toothed tigers, poor diets, and sedentary lifestyles. In the United States alone, twenty-five million adults experience heartburn daily, and more than one-third of adults experience heartburn at least once a month.[3]

The nervous system normally controls stomach-acid production; the parasympathetics stimulate stomach-acid production through the vagus nerve, a cranial nerve that connects the stomach (and other organs in the abdomen) to the brain. If a malfunction exists and the stomach gets the message to produce too much or too little digestive acid, there are two possible causes: the wrong message is being sent from the brain, or the right message is getting distorted along the vagus nerve somewhere between the brain and the stomach.

When treating a patient with heartburn or gastric reflux, I therefore consider the balance and function of the parasympathetic nervous system. Since the vagus nerve passes through a tiny opening between bones of the skull and runs very closely to vertebrae in the upper neck, I also want to ensure that none of those bones are misaligned or allowed to irritate the nerve. Either possibility should be fixable, allowing the stomach to receive the correct and uninterrupted message from the brain. Once the normal function of the vagus nerve is restored, stomach-acid production returns to normal.

Even if you've taken medications for years, your body can control itself through these sorts of physical corrections. It isn't magical healing. Healthcare is both art and science. As a doctor of chiropractic, my perspective is to consider normal or even optimal function. Even when I do the proper correction, which might include realigning bones, stimulating reflexes or acupuncture points, or adding nutrients and diets and exercise programs, I am not doing the healing. I am simply helping the body to heal itself. *Nature does the healing.*

Our bodies are self-correcting, given the opportunity, and have an amazing ability to recover from injuries and stresses. How many times before had Chris headed a soccer ball with no subsequent problems or perhaps just a mild temporary headache from the impact? Probably many. The problem is that some injuries and stresses are either so severe or affect the body so it cannot reset and heal itself. When Chris headed the heavy, wet soccer ball, the physical force to his head and neck was sufficient to misalign bones in a way that his body was unable to self-correct. Many chronic health problems originate this way. In patients whose injuries haven't healed properly or whose stresses have caught up with them, a physical, chemical, or emotional trauma that exceeded the body's ability to reset could be the cause.

The body's mastery at adapting

The other way in which malfunction happens is when the body adapts to a trauma rather than fixing it. Our bodies are programmed for survival. In order to meet life's demands, they may adapt to a problem that is not easily fixed. Mechanically, this can take place anywhere in the body and is often difficult for us to identify ourselves. A common example is how people can develop a knee, lower back, or shoulder problem following an ankle injury. Ankle sprains and strains are notorious for creating problems elsewhere that may go unnoticed for months or years. Then, when the adaptation to the original injury becomes enough of a problem itself, the person may seek help and not know what type of doctor to go to. The symptom is probably a musculoskeletal pain or limited motion, but not many doctors think functionally, i.e., they don't relate the symptom to the possibility of an earlier ankle injury. The new symptom will probably be labeled tendonitis, bursitis, or joint inflammation. Traditional treatment may be medications to control pain and inflammation or else nothing. The dysfunction goes unrecognized and therefore is not fixed.

Why do ankle sprains, when untreated, cause symptoms in the knee, lower back, or shoulder? Nerve endings, called mechano-receptors, in the joints of the feet, are triggered by the motion of body parts and then send information to the nervous system so it can coordinate the motion.

Think about normal walking. Your arms move without conscious control. When you step forward with your right leg, your left arm goes forward. That's because the nerve endings in the joints of your right foot and ankle send signals to your brain, which now knows to turn on and off specific muscles in the left shoulder as well as in the neck, lower back, and legs. The whole dance is precisely controlled and integrated by the nervous system.

But the brain requires the proper information from the nerve endings in the ankle. If bones of the ankle or foot are misaligned from an injury, nerve endings in the ligaments around the affected joints may not signal properly. When that happens, the nervous system doesn't get accurate information about stepping forward with your right foot and then doesn't coordinate other muscles to act properly in response. If the muscles of your left shoulder don't turn on and off properly when you move, it's likely you'll eventually develop a problem in your left shoulder.

Long after an ankle sprain, many of us still have misaligned joints in our ankles that cause the mechanoreceptors in the ligaments to fire improperly, thus creating problems elsewhere in the body.

The doctor's challenge is to first identify the problem in the ankle and then correct it with an adjustment to the misaligned joint. It requires knowing which bone is misaligned and in which direction and testing the muscles that surround and support the joint to make sure they are functioning properly. If they aren't, I do specific corrections to reset them and restore normal function.

Again, sometimes the body can correct its muscles so they heal properly after an injury, and sometimes it can't. Ankle sprains often leave the ankle muscles abnormally "shut off" even years later, which is one of the big reasons why ankles are frequently reinjured. Someone just steps down on it "wrong" and it gives out again. It really is unfortunate how many people are forced to limit their physical activity, sometimes for years, due to an ankle injury that didn't heal properly or that wasn't corrected so it could heal.[4]

The ankle is an amazing shock absorber. When you walk or run, the impact on the foot causes nerve endings to send information to the nervous system which should result in the facilitation or turning on of muscles that support the ankle, knee, hip, and lower back. But what happens to a knee or hip over years of extra wear and tear if the supporting muscles are not doing their jobs? It's about the same result as when a car's shock absorbers are shot; the tires and suspension take a real beating, and other parts wear out. Knees and hips can wear out prematurely, too.

People often ask if running is good or bad for you. My answer is that it all depends on how the body is functioning. Running itself is not bad for you, and it should actually be good for you. It depends on how well your shock absorbers and supporting muscles are working. If you have a malfunctioning foot from an old, unhealed injury, running could easily cause premature deterioration or even a new injury of the knee or hip.

It is so important to "make exercise your ally," which requires (1) exercising properly and (2) making sure that your body is functioning well—addressing any symptoms that your body's parts need adjustment. The second part may require you to consult with a doctor who looks at the overall function of the body and can correct and reset areas that are being affected by old injuries.

This is a whole different kind of doctoring than identifying a disease process and knowing the best medications and surgical procedure for dealing with it. And without this kind of holistic doctoring, people decline into chronic conditions much earlier in life. One of the worst things you can do is to limit your activity or compromise your lifestyle *because of an injury that may very well be correctable.*

If you have had any kind of mechanical trauma to your body and feel like you have never been the same since, or if you have experienced a mechanical injury that has created a lingering symptom or disability, consult with a doctor who does mechanical corrections. You may find that restoring normal function to your body brings life to your years and even years to your life.

Evaluating body function

How is the testing, the functional analysis, performed that reveals the dysfunction within a body and helps determine what needs to be corrected? First, here's some basic neurology: To produce motion, muscles are turned "on" or "off" by the nervous system in a process called facilitation and inhibition. In order to flex your elbow, your biceps have to be turned on (facilitated) and your triceps have to be turned off (inhibited). Without both of these reactions, you won't flex your elbow, or you will struggle doing it. It's the same when your arm swings forward when you step with the opposite leg. To swing your arm forward, the muscles that pull it back have to shut off and the muscles that pull it forward have to turn on. Since a failure of this normal neurological mechanism is going to create problems sooner or later, the ability to identify and correct it is quite valuable.

A system of manual muscle testing was developed at Johns Hopkins University in the 1940s that can be used to determine if the nervous system is functioning normally.[5] Researchers identified ways to selectively test the major muscles of the body, using biomechanics to position parts of the body and see if the patient could hold their body in certain positions against resistance. For example, if you can hold your straight arm in toward your body while a trained tester applies pressure trying to pull it out and slightly forward, it means that a specific muscle, the latissimus dorsi, is on. This muscle pulls back on the arm and pulls down on the shoulder. It has to shut off during walking to allow the arm to go forward with the opposite leg. It also has to turn on to pull back on the arm when the leg on the same side goes forward. It is a very important muscle for swimmers, but everyone uses it during normal daily activities.

Frequently muscles don't turn on and off as they should. Sometimes they are stuck on, but more often they are shut off when they shouldn't be. It can happen from an injury to the muscle itself or from a malfunction in another part of the body. It is common for an injury to abnormally shut off muscles, even years later, and create adaptations or secondary problems in the body. Muscles move bones and are necessary for normal body mechanics. Muscles support joints. What if a muscle that supports the inner border of the knee was improperly shut off for years? Not only would you have instability of your knee, but you would have premature wear and tear on the medial knee and possibly chronic pain and inflammation. If you took medication to control the pain and inflammation without correcting the muscle imbalance, you could actually be accelerating deterioration of your knee. For a knee problem, it is wise to consult with someone who approaches the problem functionally and can (1) test alignment of the knee itself, (2) test muscles that support the knee, and (3) test that the ankle is absorbing shock properly and sending the right messages to the nervous system.

Knee problems of this type are extremely common, often due to an old injury to the knee and one or more ankle sprains. So many times, people tell me they used to be very active but hardly exercise anymore because they get so sore that it feels like they are doing more harm than good. With proper testing of knee muscles and treatment, chronic knee problems can usually be helped.

A muscle that tests weak is not usually weak from a lack of exercise. Nor can it usually be corrected by exercise itself. The manual muscle test evaluates for a difference in function, or whether the muscle is turned on or off by the nervous system.[6] It does not test for muscle strength. There is a distinct difference between a muscle that tests weak because it is turned off and a muscle that is weak from fatigue or a lack of exercise.[7] When a muscle is neurologically inhibited or turned off, the muscle often exerts the same amount of force as a turned on or facilitated muscle, but the timing of its electrical activity is delayed. This delay in the firing of the electrical activity of the inhibited muscle means it fails to lock against the tester's pressure. The muscle doesn't respond instantaneously like a normal facilitated muscle. That delay is also what prevents the muscle from properly supporting the joint (such as the hip, knee, or ankle) that it is supposed to protect. It is what allows someone's ankle, knee, or lower back to "give out" suddenly if they move wrong. It creates many shoulder problems, such as when a person can't bring his arm all the way up or perhaps gets a lot of popping sounds when he tries, because the muscles aren't working together properly.

The turned-off or neurologically inhibited muscle is distinctly different from a weak muscle, even though it tests as if it is weak. Here's an analogy: If you walk into a dark room, you turn on the light. If the light didn't go on, you might check to make sure the bulb isn't burnt out. You wouldn't check the bulb if you haven't already tried the on/off switch. I look at normal muscle function in a similar way. Exercising a weak muscle is like putting in a fresh light bulb. Though strengthening the muscle may be essential, it still won't work properly unless the switch is turning it on and off. Corrections to the body reset the switches and restore the normal turning on and off of muscles. People very often reinjure themselves by trying to strengthen a muscle that is turned off. They put in a fresh light bulb and can't figure out why the light doesn't go on. They don't consider the possibility that the switch may be off. This is one of the major reasons why so many people give up on exercise or activities they love to do. But would you sell your car if you discovered the tires were wearing unevenly? Of course not. You would have an expert evaluate it and tell you what is wrong—likely an alignment problem—which you would then have corrected. Why not give your body the same consideration?

Once a muscle is turned on properly, even though it may have been off for years, exercise may still be needed, but the improvement in muscle and joint function is often dramatic once the circuitry that controls the muscle is corrected.

This sort of muscle testing is based on a system called Applied Kinesiology (AK) discovered in 1964 by Dr. George Goodheart. He expanded greatly on classical kinesiology and biomechanics (the sciences that evaluate how muscles produce motion for all human activity) by utilizing them to evaluate body function. He then used many of the procedures from chiropractic, osteopathy, acupuncture, and nutrition to correct dysfunctions in the body. His approach is to measure body function, make the appropriate correction to the body indicated by the measurement, and then remeasure to make sure that the correction was effective. This approach is used by many doctors throughout the world. Even though it is logical and sensible, it is a different way of evaluating the body and seems strange to people who don't consider a functional approach to health and disease. This approach looks at the whole person and how you function structurally, chemically, and emotionally.

Manual muscle testing is used in many different ways to monitor body function. A layperson's approach, called Touch for Health, enables nonprofessionals to do basic muscle testing to assess for imbalances and then use various reflexes to balance the energy.

Applied Kinesiology is performed by health professionals, who use manual muscle testing in conjunction with other standard diagnostic tests. An Applied Kinesiology approach to evaluating a chronic knee problem evaluates the person with the knee problem, not just the knee. It includes a thorough health history, including past injuries, diet, and exercise. It involves orthopedic and neurological tests for both structure and function, possibly X-rays or MRIs—whatever is necessary to look at the big picture. Biomechanical assessment and functional tests of the pelvis, knee, and ankle then identify specific areas to correct, which may then improve the function of the knee.

Mechanical dysfunction is common, and it is the underlying cause of many chronic symptoms as well as increased wear and tear that accelerates aging and brings on chronic disease. A great deal of mechanical dysfunction can be identified and then corrected—or at least minimized.

Summary of Key Points

1. Holistic healthcare strives to treat the person who has the problem.

2. In healthcare, "one size does not fit all."

3. Successful outcomes require matching the treatment to the patient.

4. If symptoms develop following mechanical trauma to the body, think mechanical! Consult with a doctor who does mechanical corrections to the body (probably a doctor of chiropractic or osteopathy).

5. Nature does the healing.

6. The body is a self-correcting mechanism.
    a. If symptoms persist following an injury or trauma to the body, the body may be unable to self-correct.
    b. If a new part of the body develops symptoms after injury or trauma to a seemingly unrelated part, it may be an adaptation. This is the origin of many chronic health problems.
    In either case, it is wise to consult a doctor who analyzes body function and corrects dysfunction.

7. Muscles turn on and off during normal activity.

8. The turning on and off of muscles is controlled by the nervous system.

9. Injuries often result in muscles being turned off abnormally, leaving joints unsupported and unprotected. Muscles move bones.

10. Muscles that are turned off can be identified through manual muscle testing because they test as if they are weak.

11. For chronic problems following an injury, have someone (probably an Applied Kinesiologist) evaluate for abnormal turning off of muscles. Correct, if necessary.

12. Make exercise your ally by exercising correctly and having your body parts working properly.

Correcting the Faulty Mechanisms

How Pete's gastroesophageal reflux disease was due to anatomical-biomechanical factors that were modifiable and how Richard's low-back pain and golf game were both helped by correcting a specific problem in his neck

We've seen how mechanical dysfunction in the body creates a variety of common symptoms. In this section, you'll look behind the symptoms of a common disease, gastroesophageal reflux disease, to the mechanisms that create it and then to the corrections that can be made. Gastroesophageal reflux disease (GERD) is a common chronic disease that is often due to anatomical and biomechanical factors that can by modified.

Later in this section is another example of a faulty mechanism. We'll show how a person's low-back pain *and* golf game were improved by correcting a specific problem in his upper neck.

The second-most-important muscle in the body

Pete has been one of my patients for over twenty years. At eighty, he is healthy and vibrant. He plays tennis several times a week, is active in his work and in civic organizations, and serves on the board of directors of a local hospital. Pete got the message years ago about the value of taking care of his health. He is an inspiration and a tribute to healthy aging. We have worked together to keep his body functioning as well as possible and to provide the most appropriate nutritional supplements.

Within the last year, Pete began having severe symptoms of acid reflux. When he came in to the office with this complaint, I did some mechanical corrections on him that would influence his body's control of acid reflux.

On his following visit, several weeks later, he began by telling me, in amazement, that the acid reflux had been totally absent since I worked on it. Naturally, we were both thrilled at the positive outcome. But there was more to the story.

He had been evaluated for this problem at the hospital a few months previously. They scoped his esophagus and stomach, ran other tests, and gave him a name for what he had: gastroesophageal reflux disease (GERD). He was advised that his only course of action was to take medication and to hope it would not turn into esophageal cancer. The medication helped with the burning, but there wasn't any change in the reflux itself until I worked on it.

For all the high-technology diagnostic testing, no treatment had been offered to Pete except to take a pill. There was no guidance and no follow-up, and only minimal help from the pill. He was struck by the contrast of how my physical treatment for the problem had helped it enormously.

In evaluating patients, I get as much data as I can about their health. The first step in treatment is identifying the malfunction. Extensive interviews of the patient, functional testing, scanning and diagnostic imaging techniques, and laboratory testing are extremely valuable tools in determining what mechanism in the body needs correction.

And once you find out what is wrong, you have to fix it or improve body function. That is where procedures from Applied Kinesiology, chiropractic, osteopathy, craniosacral therapy, and acupuncture really shine because they actually improve the function of the body.

Pete is not alone in experiencing the strengths and weaknesses of traditional Western medicine. While it often provides the most advanced diagnoses, it doesn't always offer the best treatment available. No one has all the answers for all health problems. But as a patient, before you resort to taking pharmaceutical drugs forever, at least consider the mechanisms that underlie your symptoms and question whether the function of those mechanisms could be improved.

Using gastric reflux, let's look at normal function and consider the symptoms as evidence of some function that has gone wrong but is potentially fixable. The stomach produces digestive acid and enzymes that are essential to break down food. If you don't produce enough acid, you can't break down your food properly and you can become deficient in nutrients that would be absorbed into your bloodstream from your food. The acid-base (pH) balance in your body can even shift, causing joint stiffness and calcium deposits.

It was recently found that people who take medications to suppress production of gastric acid have a higher incidence of pneumonia, presumably because the drugs compromise the protective function of the acid, in which it kills bacteria entering the stomach.[8] Your stomach acid is important for normal physiology and function. In the beautiful and grand design of the body, the stomach's protective lining prevents the acid from destroying the stomach itself. The body is built to withstand the very potent acid, as long as the acid stays in the stomach.

The esophagus, the tube that carries food from the mouth to the stomach, does not have a protective lining to prevent the acid from eating away at it. Therefore, acid that gets up into the esophagus can produce the burning symptoms of gastroesophageal reflux disease and can be destructive to the esophagus over time.

The body normally keeps acid in the stomach by the function of the diaphragm, the muscle that separates the chest and abdominal cavities and contains the esophageal sphincter, the all-important barrier between the stomach and the esophagus. It is the tone of the diaphragm muscle and the esophageal sphincter that maintains the barrier and keeps acid in the stomach and out of the esophagus.

Therefore, if you have a problem with acid rising up into the esophagus, it makes sense to consider that those muscles may not be doing their jobs. Looked at in this way, as a potential faulty mechanism, it becomes logical to seek healthcare that promotes the normal function of those muscles.

Medical textbooks note that hiatal hernia symptoms such as acid reflux result from muscle laxity or weakness around the esophageal sphincter. Many people, including Pete, respond to correcting the dysfunction of the diaphragm muscle and to a visceral manipulation that pulls down on the stomach, which is otherwise being pushed up through the opening into the esophagus. Once the muscle imbalance is corrected, the esophageal sphincter can do its normal job of preventing stomach acid from rising into the esophagus. The acid can do its vital task of breaking down food in the stomach without causing problems, and the person's digestive process can return to normal.

Correcting a dysfunctioning muscle makes sense. It's non-invasive, holistic, and can impact a patient's life in broader ways than just solving the mechanical problem. What doesn't make sense is the standard first line of treatment that millions receive for this problem, which is to take medications to reduce acid production.

It makes no sense to assume that everyone with heartburn and reflux symptoms has excess acid production. On the contrary, many of these people don't have too much acid. The problem is that the acid is in the wrong place—up in the esophagus where it doesn't belong. Rather than a chemical problem (too much acid production), it's likely to be a mechanical problem with a muscle, a problem that can be corrected.

To further understand the mechanism, let's look at the diaphragm. Like the biceps or triceps, the diaphragm is a muscle that can be weak from a lack of exercise. Compare the difference between the activity of a sedentary person who breathes all day and night in a shallow manner with the workout the diaphragm gets during physical exercise. Any activity that forces you to breathe harder and deeper is exercising the diaphragm muscle.

The diaphragm can also be inhibited or shut off by the nervous system due to an injury or other malfunction in the body. However, the diaphragm is special; I consider it second only to the heart as the most important muscle in the body. The diaphragm not only increases oxygen levels in the brain and throughout the body, it also pumps the acupuncture energy that flows through your meridian system.

When you have a sluggish diaphragm muscle, you are prone to fatigue, mental symptoms such as poor concentration, unclear thinking, failing memory, and other symptoms in addition to gastric reflux. Imagine what it does to your mental function if your brain receives 20 or 30 percent less oxygen than optimum, year after year, due to a weak or inhibited diaphragm muscle. This sustained oxygen deficit could result in a premature decline in brain function, which is exactly what happens to many people. A normally functioning diaphragm muscle, along with proper breathing and regular exercise to keep the muscle strong, can make a critical difference in slowing the aging process.

Weakness of the diaphragm is extremely common. Although not everyone with a weak diaphragm muscle develops a hiatal hernia (where a portion of the stomach protrudes up through the esophageal opening), the frequency of hiatal hernias increases with age. However, the exact frequency is not known since not everyone has been tested for it. But heartburn, the primary symptom, is a consistent problem for about 15 percent of the population worldwide and affects at least 40 percent of the population in the United States on a monthly basis.[9]

Good diaphragm function is important for your health and vitality. Antioxidants, found in fruits and vegetables, can be quite helpful. But the best antioxidant is oxygen itself. If you improve your body's ability to deliver oxygen to its own tissues, you reduce oxidative stress and tissue damage throughout your body and slow the decline in body function that occurs with aging.

While I recommend that many of my patients take antioxidant nutrients, I definitely want to optimize the vital function of the diaphragm muscle. I test for it in almost every patient, regardless of their symptoms, because I know that by correcting it, I have a good chance of helping their digestion, mental function, and overall energy and well-being.

How can the function of the diaphragm be improved? The first step, as with any malfunctioning muscle, is to identify what could be inhibiting or weakening the muscle. With the diaphragm, there are common patterns of weakness. The nerves that stimulate the diaphragm exit the spine in two areas, the neck or mid-cervical spine and the lower thoracic spine, where the ribcage ends. If these spinal areas are misaligned or fixated (failing to move properly), there can be a reflex inhibition, or weakness, of the diaphragm.

Other common faulty mechanisms can affect the diaphragm. If the rib cage is not moving freely on either side, usually from past injury, the motion of the diaphragm can be limited. A common pelvic or lower-back misalignment creates a torquing in the body that limits diaphragm motion. If the cranial bones are misaligned or limited in their normal respiratory motion, this can prevent a person from breathing deeply. An important lower-back supporting muscle, the psoas, attaches indirectly to the diaphragm. A common imbalance of this muscle can also compromise the diaphragm. Many people with low-back problems have an imbalance of this muscle.

All of these are switches that commonly disturb the normal function of the diaphragm. To obtain normal function of the diaphragm, a healthcare provider has to determine which biomechanics are impeding its normal function. Treatment then entails manipulation or adjustments to specific areas of the spine that affect nerves leading to the diaphragm, or the correction of other muscle imbalances as well as a manipulation to the stomach itself.

Consider what frequently happens to the stomach over a lifetime. As we age, our shoulders and upper back can become increasingly hunched over. In mechanical terms, thoracic kyphosis increases, or we get more kyphotic. Try this: hunch over for a moment and try to take a deep breath. It's difficult, because there is no room for your diaphragm to move when you are in that position. If you were constantly in that position, you'd never be able to take a deep breath and, of course, your brain would receive less oxygen. Furthermore, in that position your stomach is compressed up into your diaphragm, putting extra pressure on the esophageal sphincter and challenging its ability to keep the contents of your stomach out of your esophagus. Now sit or stand up straight and take in a deep breath. Not only can you inhale more oxygen, but you might even feel your head clear immediately.

Let's take it a step further. If you ate a large meal while hunched over, your full and expanded stomach, which is being compressed by your position, has nowhere to go but up into your diaphragm. If your diaphragm and esophageal sphincter are weak, the upward pressure of your stomach can force a portion of the stomach or its contents into the esophagus, causing gastric reflux and even a hiatal hernia.

From a functional point of view, it is easy to understand how poor posture, a full stomach, and a weak diaphragm muscle can create gastric reflux. The manipulation of the stomach performed by a health professional involves gently pulling down on the stomach to reduce its upward pressure on the diaphragm while the patient breathes a certain way. This correction can reduce the pressure and weakness of the diaphragm and is most effective if the patient can also improve muscle function, straighten their posture, and learn to breathe more deeply. A chiropractor can help a person improve their posture through spinal corrections and by treating the extensor muscles that help hold the body upright. In addition to spinal correction, I teach people several stretching and breathing exercises and encourage more physical activity to activate the diaphragm.

One reasons for the recent increase in diaphragm-related problems in younger people is that a sedentary lifestyle generally means more sitting, poor posture, and shallow breathing. Like any other muscle, the diaphragm must be used. I turn on the switch through treatment, and the patient puts in a fresh bulb by breathing properly and exercising. If we each do our part, the light goes on. For most people, a couple of visits are sufficient to correct a diaphragm imbalance. They may need to have it checked or fixed periodically to maintain the correction, especially if they don't exercise, if they overeat and lie down too soon after eating, or if they are under a lot of stress. For some older people who are already quite hunched over, I may not be able to fully correct the problem, but usually I can maintain some significant amount of improvement through periodic treatments.

Stress can adversely affect the diaphragm in several ways. In stressful situations, you naturally tighten up. You breathe less deeply and sometimes feel tightness in your chest. I frequently remind people to breathe deeply during stressful times or even when working intensely in a stationary position. A more extreme example of diaphragm tightness is caused by a physical trauma. Most of us have had the wind knocked out of us from a fall or a physical injury, which is a good reminder of what a spastic diaphragm feels like.

Emotional traumas and stresses can have a similar tightening effect on the diaphragm. On a deeper level, chronic stress can really upset the diaphragm. The body's sphincter muscles, such as the esophageal sphincter, are controlled by the autonomic nervous system. The sympathetic nerves tighten the sphincters, while the parasympathetic nerves relax them. When you are exhausted from constant encounters with saber-toothed tigers, your sympathetic nervous system (which enables the fight-or-flee response) is depleted and may be unable to maintain the normal tone of the sphincters. This laxity of the sphincter then predisposes you to gastric reflux. If you are chronically stressed, adjustments and corrections that selectively stimulate specific parts of the nervous system are useful, as is taking specific vitamins and nutrients that will provide the building blocks to rebuild exhausted parts and functions of the body. And of course you must commit yourself to lifestyle changes that reduce the effects of the saber-toothed tiger on your body so your body can heal itself.

The holistic approach involves both you and your healthcare provider working to create more balance in your nervous system and to rebuild depleted or exhausted areas. This is a far different approach to chronic health problems than traditional Western medicine's approach of replacing whatever it is the body can no longer do, such as prescribing hormones if a person's glands can no longer produce enough, or removing or replacing an organ that no longer functions properly.

In the earlier example, Pete was discouraged when his medical doctor offered no hope of improving his reflux problem. He was told that the reflux would continue to worsen and that if it turned into esophageal cancer, he'd probably be dead within six months. Clearly, that dismal prognosis did not consider treating Pete with the aim of modifying the faulty mechanisms which created the problem in the first place and thereby allowing the body to control and heal itself.

The widespread effects of mechanical dysfunction

Richard, a patient in his fifties, was having muscle spasms in his lower back. The only thing he had been doing differently was to play more golf than he had previously. In mentioning his back spasms to other golfers, he was surprised to learn that many of them experienced similar pain. I knew I could very likely help him because several patterns of mechanical imbalance are common among golfers, and they are usually correctable.

One of the most common mechanical imbalances is a fixation, which is a lack of normal motion of the vertebrae in the upper neck that causes a weakness or inhibition of specific lower back muscles. That lower back weakness then causes a secondary spasm of the opposing muscles in the back, even though the source of the problem is in the neck. The ligaments around the vertebrae in the upper neck contain an enormous number of mechanoreceptors, nerve endings that send information to the brain, informing it about one's head position. The accuracy of this information is critical to coordination and balance as well as the proper turning on and off of certain muscles. These nerve endings even affect the jaw muscles and, in some people, can lead to TMJ (temporomandibular joint) problems. In short, the input to the brain from joint receptors in the upper neck is quite significant. Correcting a mechanical problem in the neck can eliminate back spasms and sometimes even improve golf performance.

To demonstrate this to Richard, I asked him to stand up and focus his eyes on the upper corner of the room, where the ceiling meets the intersecting walls. I asked him to point to that spot. He raised his arm and pointed to the spot. I then instructed him to drop his arm and then repeat the procedure, but with his eyes closed, using his visual memory of the location of the spot where the ceiling meets the intersecting wall. With his eyes shut, he raised his arm and pointed to the spot. I told him then to open his eyes. We both observed that his "eyes closed" pointing was up and to the right of the true location by quite a bit. If it had been right on, as it should be, it would have meant that his brain was probably receiving accurate messages from his upper neck. And when he hit a golf ball, it would be more likely to go where he thought he visualized it going instead of off to one side. That brought a laugh from Richard, who was convinced his golf game was beyond repair.

I proceeded to do specific testing on Richard, specifically a manual muscle test of his gluteus maximus muscles to see if they were properly supporting his lower back and legs. For the test, he lay face down on the examination table and then bent his left knee and raised his thigh into the air. I then pushed down on his thigh and asked him to resist my pressure. With just a small amount of pressure, I was able to push Richard's leg down. Simply raising the leg into the test position created some pain and spasm in his lower back, and he even commented on how weak it felt. Getting the same result from testing his right leg, I concluded that both of Richard's gluteus maximus muscles were being inhibited or shut off by his nervous system. Even though the muscles tested weak and felt weak to Richard, the muscles themselves were probably normal. Richard exercises regularly and has exceptional muscle tone. The muscles actually felt fine to the touch; they simply were not turning on properly. To use the earlier analogy, the light bulb was fine, but the switch was off. Those muscles are innocent victims. With the switch turned off, those gluteus maximus muscles cannot properly support the lower back.

Like Richard, anyone with this problem would experience a chronically weak lower back, often worsened by attempts to strengthen it. With this particular imbalance, people also commonly experience tight hamstring muscles due to the failure of the gluteus maximus muscles to pull down the back of the pelvis as they normally would. The gluteus maximus muscles even support the outside of the knees, so people lacking that support sometimes develop lateral knee problems and iliotibial band syndromes.

Bilateral gluteus maximus weakness is fairly common and, as you can see, creates several different symptoms. Of great significance is that this lower back muscle weakness is usually caused by a fixation of the vertebrae in the upper neck, whereby the mechanoreceptors in the ligaments around the joints send erroneous information, such as telling Richard's nervous system that his head is level when it really isn't. Then his body must compensate for the faulty information by setting up other mechanisms in the attempt to preserve balance and coordination.

After the muscle test, I then evaluated the vertebrae of Richard's upper neck, carefully feeling for proper alignment as well as the normal motion that should be present in the joints between the vertebrae. Upon finding the specific location of the vertebral fixation, I corrected it by a painless adjustment in which I placed one hand on each vertebra and gave a light, precise thrusting motion on the two vertebrae to get them unstuck. Immediately after the correction, I retested the gluteus maximus muscles. On this second testing, Richard was able to effortlessly hold each thigh up in the air with no strain or spasm in his lower back. After the adjustment, the muscles were being properly turned on by Richard's nervous system because the ligaments of the upper neck were sending proper signals to the brain. With those muscles now functioning normally, I fully expected his lower back to feel much better, which it did almost immediately.

Next, I asked him to do the "pointing test" again. Richard stood up and focused on the corner of the room. He lined up his finger with the corner, first with his eyes open. After dropping his arm to the side, he closed his eyes and did it again but with his eyes closed. He was astounded to observe that he could now line it up perfectly. I told him there was a very good chance he would now find himself hitting the golf ball more where he visualized it going rather than to either side of his mental image. Yes, when given the opportunity, our bodies are simply amazing in their ability to function well.

The body is a system of self-correcting mechanisms that try to rebuild, repair, and restore balance. But so often the body can't correct itself because of past injuries that haven't healed properly or from a lifestyle that damages and depletes the body, depriving it of the opportunity to heal. As a practitioner of complementary and alternative medicine, I give my patients every opportunity to help their bodies heal themselves. Nature heals, given the chance. Unfortunately, many of us just never give it the chance. We are taught to think that medications heal, and that's all there is. In reality, medications kill off invading microbes, replace body functions, and modify symptoms. They sometimes allow the body to heal, but they don't do the healing, just as I don't. My role, and the role of any healthcare provider, should be to provide therapeutic interventions that allow and encourage nature to do its own powerful healing work.

Summary of Key Points

1. Although the mainstream management of GERD is primarily chemical, the faulty mechanisms in the body that create GERD are primarily anatomical and biomechanical.

2. GERD symptoms may not be from an excess of acid production but from the acid being in the wrong place; for example, acid getting up into the esophagus, which does not have the same protective lining as the stomach.

3. The phrase, "There is no treatment other than medication," may really mean, "I don't know of anything that could help this besides medication."

4. While TWM may excel in high-tech diagnostic testing, CAM often shines in the realm of effective treatment.

5. The diaphragm is the second-most-important muscle in the body, second only to the heart.

6. GERD symptoms can be reduced or eliminated by restoring normal function of the diaphragm and esophageal sphincter, along with a program of exercise and proper breathing.

7. *Where* one experiences a symptom is not necessarily where the problem lies. (For example, Richard's lower back pain was caused by a malfunction in his upper neck.)

8. Mechanoreceptors in the joints of the upper neck can affect balance, coordination, and muscle tone throughout the body.

9. Chiropractic treatments can restore normal mechanoreceptor activity to malfunctioning joints.

Improving Health versus Treating Disease

What it means to treat the person who has the back pain

Esther is an amazing, spry lady of eighty-three years. Besides raising a family, Esther had a very active career in the field of education. She first came to my office complaining that she was now limited in her activities due to extensive stiffness and pain in her back. She had recently been through a period of stress including a bout with colon cancer that required surgery to remove a section of her large intestine. She tolerated the surgery well and was free of the cancer, but she had developed increasing back pain and disability in the following year. Due to the severity of her pain, doctors had X-rays taken to determine the condition of her spine. As would be expected in the spine of someone who has lived a very active eighty-plus years, the X-rays showed considerable degeneration of the vertebrae and discs in her lower spine.

Although her doctors informed Esther that she had severe degenerative joint disease and osteoarthritis, I hesitate to use those terms because they are misleading. The terms sound as though she had acquired a disease for which there is no cure. Four orthopedic surgeons informed Esther that her disease was inoperable and that nothing could be done other than taking medication to dull the pain. Esther told me how extremely disheartening it was to be told that no treatment was available and that, indeed, her condition would worsen and she would eventually be crippled and unable to walk.

Fortunately, she did not blindly accept this prognosis. She has a great love for life, for nature, for people, and for intellectual stimulation, and she is quite resourceful. So she took it upon herself to explore other options for treating her condition. Even as a layperson, she knew of things she could do to help herself: improve her diet and take supplements, exercise, and ... she could find another doctor, one who would work with her and look for solutions.

Esther was referred to me and recognized immediately that I saw her problem differently than her other doctors had. I looked at the same X-rays but from the perspective that they showed not a static picture but rather an ongoing process with variables that could be altered. In the extensive health history I took, I discovered great significance in her past injuries, her blood tests, her likes and dislikes, her diet and exercise, her stresses, and even her dental history. I did many functional tests that had not previously been performed on her, and I concluded that while I probably could not change the appearance of her X-rays, I had discovered a number of areas we could approach that might help her spine function better, even though the deterioration was quite advanced.

The spectrum of structure and function

Before I discuss the things that Esther and I did to improve her health, consider a spectrum, with structure on one end and function on the other. My approach to health includes both but emphasizes function. I see the same severity of deterioration on Esther's X-rays as anyone else. But I see it in the context of an ongoing process. My analysis of the X-ray of the vertebrae led me to note these issues:

- The spine has deteriorated. The first question is this: Are the muscles that should support her discs and vertebrae turning on and off properly?

- There are signs of inflammation and calcium deposition. I'll investigate to see if anything can be done to improve her body's regulation of this osteoarthritic process.

- There is extensive misalignment of the vertebrae and the indication of multiple discs bulging. I will determine if the degree of misalignment of the vertebrae and protrusion of the discs against the nerves can be reduced.

This amount of spinal wear and tear means that the shock-absorbing mechanisms in Esther's feet have not been working well for some time. This can probably be improved.

Aside from the spinal X-rays, I look at the *person* who has the back pain. My treatment is informed by what I learn from the patient's health history:

- Esther had had several very stressful years preceding the pain. From this, I theorize that her adrenal glands may have become

67

depleted during that period. If so, they may be deficient in their production of anti-inflammatory chemicals, a deficiency that contributes to more pain and stiffness.

- Esther's back pain intensified after her colon surgery. With this information, I decide to determine if some of her pain could be referred from internal organs or caused by adhesions in the abdominal cavity.

By "thinking outside the box" about the body's function and not just about its structure, all of these become reasonable avenues to investigate. If any or all of them are contributing to her pain and can be improved, Esther's pain and stiffness could be reduced. Does this mean I have a magic cure for her osteoarthritis or degenerative joint disease? Of course not. It just means that those "diseases" that her other doctors say she *has* are really *conditions* that are modifiable if you can alter the mechanisms that create and control them.

Together, Esther and I can't undo or reverse much of the wear and tear that has accumulated over eighty years. If I could have treated her thirty or forty years ago to improve her alignment, muscle balance, and shock absorption, she would likely have much less spinal deterioration today. I have seen many spinal X-rays of people in their eighties. Fortunately, they don't all exhibit as much wear and tear as Esther's. Yet there are people in their sixties and seventies with as much or more degeneration. Spinal degeneration really depends on your genetic makeup, on your inherent strengths and weaknesses, and on what the events of life do to you.

The contrast between structure and function becomes evident when you see spinal X-rays that show as much or more deterioration than Esther's in people who are experiencing very little pain or stiffness. Then again, it's not unusual to see spinal X-rays showing much less deterioration in people who experience a tremendous amount of back pain and stiffness. And in practical terms, it means that the amount of deterioration on someone's spinal X-rays doesn't necessarily doom them to a life of pain and disability.

The point is that while the X-rays provide a good look at structure, structure is not the whole health picture. Rather than being the end of the analysis, the question becomes, as Esther's example shows, how to get that existing structure to function as well as possible in spite of its limitations.

Modifying a degenerative process

For any degenerative process, I consider three possible degrees of modifying it. First, can the process be slowed? Second, can the process be stopped? Third, can the process be reversed? To accomplish any of these is a victory, and I consider as many mechanisms as possible to modify the process.

Using Esther's spine as an example, it is unlikely that the degeneration can be reversed in a major way at her age. It is very likely, however, that the degenerative process could be slowed down and maybe even stopped by improving the function of various mechanisms. This becomes a real starting point for working with many chronic conditions.

How did I go about improving the function of Esther's body? Well, in summary, I literally worked on her body from head to toe, inside and out. I treated her cranial bones and her feet and just about everything in between, including advising her to take nutritional supplements.

I'll start with the spine itself. Spinal discs work like cushions between the vertebrae and help to preserve the size of the openings that the nerves travel through as they exit the spine. Over time, as the compression of gravity takes its toll, these discs typically become thinner and tend to bulge out from their sides. And like any other tissues in the body that weaken with age, they become less resilient.

Several biomechanical factors can either speed up or slow down the discs' degenerative process. One is that the discs themselves receive very little blood supply after the age of twelve or so. They receive nutrients and eliminate waste products via fluid exchange from the ligaments around them and from the vertebrae above and below. Motion stimulates this process. In other words, when you move one way and compress a disc on one side, it is sucking in a fresh supply of nutrients; when you move the other way, it is squeezing out waste products, eliminating the garbage. This process, called imbibition, helps to maintain the disc as living, healthy tissue.

Therefore, if two vertebrae become stuck, fixated, and fail to move properly, circulation to and from the disc between them becomes compromised. The "normal" deterioration of the disc over time accelerates, and the disc can wear out prematurely. The converse of this is that good alignment and freedom of motion of the vertebrae in the spine can play a huge role in extending the life of your discs. The human body loves motion, but the parts have to be working properly to fully receive the benefits. This is why I wish I could have treated Esther when she was in her forties or fifties. I would have worked to improve the alignment of the vertebrae and to eliminate the fixations in her spine, helping to slow the degeneration of the discs. Even in her eighties, it's not too late, however, to work to preserve the discs that she has left.

Another biomechanical factor that directly affects discs is that muscles move bones. A major lower back muscle, the psoas, attaches directly to the vertebrae and the discs of the lower spine. It is critical that the right and left psoas muscles pull equally, in a balanced manner. Recall the discussion in chapter 4 of how muscles normally turn on and off and how that is controlled by the nervous system. It is common for one of the psoas muscles to be inhibited or turned off. If you have this problem, it means that whenever you walk or even move, there are asymmetric forces working on your spine. Very simply, the vertebrae and discs are pulled away from the side of the inhibited psoas and toward the opposite side. The opposite psoas also can become shortened, or hypertonic, due to the lack of opposition from the inhibited one. When I first examined Esther, her left psoas, which was tight, tested as being on. Her right one was clearly turned off and tested as if it was quite weak. It was simply unable to properly support the right side of her spine.

I could only speculate as to how long she may have been walking around with that imbalance of her psoas muscles creating asymmetry in her lower back. In treatment of Esther, this muscle imbalance was one of the first things I worked to correct. I wanted those muscles to be pulling equally so the more she walked and moved, the more her body was pulling her spine into better alignment.

Exercise is an opportunity for the body to self-correct, *as long as the switches are working properly*. However, if the switches are off and the muscles aren't supporting the structure, exercise can increase wear and tear and increase the chance of further injury. Maintaining the normal function of the nervous system is a fundamental part of taking care of your body. It is healthcare, and it serves a whole different role than the traditional medical approach. It isn't treating disease; it is improving health!

Let's return to how I corrected that muscle imbalance in Esther's lower back. Knowing that something was "turning off" her right psoas muscle, I identified two specific areas which were causing her nervous system to inhibit that muscle. One was a problem with her right ankle, and the other a misalignment of a vertebra in her neck. The neck required a chiropractic adjustment to correct the misalignment. The ankle was also treated with adjustments to realign the bones and procedures to reset the ankle-supporting muscles. Several "turned off" ankle muscles took some work to correct because she had sprained each ankle many years ago and they never fully healed. Once the foot and ankle muscles were turned back on, I gave her some strengthening exercises.

To maintain the corrections in her unstable ankles and improve her shock absorption, I had her fitted with custom orthotics (inserts in her shoes to support her arches and provide proper alignment). Mechanoreceptors, the nerve endings in the joints of the feet, send information to the nervous system to turn on muscles that support us in standing and walking. Because Esther's right ankle was not signaling properly, her nervous system was not getting the message to turn on her right psoas muscle. I'm sure other muscles were also affected by the ankle problem and were probably corrected in the process. The normal function of the joints of the feet and ankles is critical to the health of the rest of the body.

I also did adjustments appropriate to Esther's condition to correct fixations and misalignments in her lower spine and pelvis. As we proceeded with those corrections, her pain reduced dramatically.

It isn't practical to take an MRI to look at the discs after each treatment, and I don't know if the discs would immediately look any different even if we could see them. But I do know that the muscles were functioning better and that Esther had less pain and stiffness, which probably means the nerves were less irritated.

One goal is to facilitate a change in the patient's symptoms. And if you can accomplish that without medication or other intervention, it means you must be influencing whatever is creating the symptoms. A positive change in the symptoms is reinforcement that you are influencing the cause of the symptoms. But sometimes, particularly with chronic problems, the symptoms don't change immediately with the treatment. Accepting that, it becomes necessary to formulate a treatment strategy that has the greatest chance of influencing what you think is creating or perpetuating the symptoms. You proceed with your treatment, and you support it as much as possible with the right diet, exercise, nutritional supplements—and a positive outlook.

Your triad of health: structural, chemical, and emotional

When you're faced with a healthcare condition, just keep an open mind, consider many possibilities, and address each one, taking them one at a time. We are all structural, chemical, and emotional beings—the triad of health. If you suffer from a chronic health problem, there is almost always some imbalance or malfunction on two or three sides of the triad, even though the symptoms may be on only one side.

Anyone who looked at Esther's spine as the totality of her back pain would perceive it purely as a structural problem. Yet it is ironic that prior to seeing me the only treatment offered to her was medication, which stems from the chemical side of the triad.

Let's look at Esther's back pain in relation to the health triad. Her pain has a structural component, which includes the spinal degeneration; the vertebral fixations; misalignments in the neck, pelvis, and ankle; as well as some muscle imbalance. It has an emotional component as well, as it would for anyone who has experienced chronic pain and disability. Fortunately, Ester had a very positive attitude about her situation. The chemical component includes many aspects of how the body regulates its own inflammation, joint health, pain, and even mood. The joint deterioration alone encompasses many modifiable factors, including levels of protein, calcium, and other minerals, along with the acid/base balance. Protein levels, so critical for the health of joint surfaces, are dependent not just on the protein one eats but also on how well food is digested by enzymes from the stomach and pancreas and how well the small intestine absorbs it. Each of these possible malfunctions commonly contributes to premature degeneration of joints. Furthermore, the malfunctions can often be corrected through diet and supplements and by restoring balance within the nervous system to control normal digestion.

It's not just "You are what you eat"

Digestion is a factor in many seemingly unrelated health issues. Here's why: The parasympathetic nerves stimulate normal digestion, while sympathetic nerves inhibit it. Too-frequent activation of the sympathetic nervous system by the "saber-toothed tiger" decreases our ability to properly digest food. So under frequent stress, we often end up feeling bloated after a meal and over time can become deficient in protein and other nutrients. You could eat plenty of protein and still be protein-deficient because you are not digesting it properly.

If good digestion were common, millions of people would not be complaining of heartburn. Improving the function of peoples' digestive systems can take some work, but it can usually be accomplished. One solution is to stimulate the parasympathetic nervous system through cranial bone treatment. This stimulates the cranial nerves, which then enhance normal digestion. Other chiropractic approaches often stimulate these nerves by adjustments to the upper neck. Sometimes I have patients temporarily take enzyme supplements while we are working to improve their body's production of its own enzymes. Accompanying this, I educate people about stress and encourage many "de-stressing" activities to reduce the constant activation of the sympathetic nerves. The end product is more balance and harmony within the nervous system.

Protein deficiency is common among people who have joint problems. Even when a person's blood-protein levels are within the normal range, the protein levels can be significantly less that optimal. For patients with less than optimal levels, I change their diet to ensure they are getting good quantities of quality protein and not interfering with its digestion by poor food combining. (For example, the body uses a different mixture of enzymes to digest proteins and carbohydrates. If your digestion is already compromised, it is best to not consume proteins and concentrated carbohydrates in the same meal.) I also work on improving digestion by treating their body and stimulating the normal digestive process.

"You are what you eat" is only partially correct. A more accurate phrase is "You are what you absorb." If you don't digest and absorb your food well, it can't contribute nutritional building blocks to your body. I commonly treat patients' small intestine to improve absorption of nutrients to help their joint problems. To do this, I try to stimulate the nerves that go directly to that organ from the central nervous system. For the small intestine, I stimulate specific vertebrae in the lower thoracic spine. I might also consider certain nutrients that favor production of the specific neurotransmitters that I want to increase. For example, I would advise the person to increase their choline intake by eating eggs (egg yolks are a good source of choline) to encourage a greater production of acetylcholine, a chemical that helps relay messages between nerve cells throughout the parasympathetics and part of the sympathetics. I would treat specific reflexes that stimulate the blood supply *to* the lymphatic drainage *from* the small intestine as well as specific acupuncture points that can normalize the energy patterns of the small intestine. I might also have a person take specific nutrients to improve the absorption abilities and function of the small intestine and have them discontinue certain foods or combinations of foods that don't agree with their small intestine or some other part of the body.

As odd as it sounds, your small intestine is one of your links to the outside world. Most of what comes into your body does so by absorption through the small intestine. If you eat bad foods or foods you may be sensitive to or allergic to, your small intestine will react by reducing absorption, perhaps for survival reasons. It is likely that the small intestine even contains emotional receptors, which brings another whole dimension to our understanding of its importance. When we say we have a "gut feeling," it may be true. It doesn't mean that every "gut feeling" is accurate, but we do feel with our gut. There is a lot of information being relayed between the gut and the brain and vice versa.

In short, the correction of protein digestion and absorption is systematic and can help you by slowing deterioration of your joints. A variety of treatment procedures can be done to actually improve the function of a vital organ such as the small intestine and subsequently improve your overall nutritional status because of better absorption of the nutrients in your diet and supplements.

To summarize, if you can get all three sides of the triad of health—your body's structure, chemistry, and emotions—working together and for you, instead of against you, you can usually make progress in improving your health. Esther has made it a point to exercise regularly, and it was not always easy for her. She derives considerable benefit from it, and it ultimately helps the whole triad. Emotionally, she feels good doing it; she knows she is actively caring for health. Structurally, it is good for her bones, muscles, discs, and flexibility. Chemically, it helps her body burn fat and produce good chemicals, such as prostaglandins, which are anti-inflammatory and help her emotional state.

As doctor and patient, we have a partnership in helping to improve her health. She exercises, eats a healthful diet, takes supplements, and maintains periodic appointments with me. I work to identify imbalances in her system and make corrections that promote harmony in her body, allowing the healing power of nature to do its work. On every visit, I study her posture and closely watch her walk. I observe for any structural or muscle imbalance that may be a key to what would best be treated on that visit. With my fingers, I feel areas on her skull, neck, abdomen, legs, and feet. I evaluate how her feet and ankles line up. Knowing that her legs are anatomically the same length (and not everyone's are), any measurable difference, from right to left, is a *functional* leg-length difference and can be evened out through gentle correction that realigns the pelvis. I usually do several cranial corrections to stimulate the parasympathetic nervous system and to balance the tension on her spine by affecting its attachments to the cranial bones. I work on her diaphragm muscle and do some visceral manipulation on her abdomen. I stimulate acupuncture points on her knees and ankles and correct any other misaligned vertebrae with chiropractic adjustments to help her spine and discs.

When Esther stands up again after being treated, I closely reexamine her posture and gait. There is almost always a significant and observable improvement in the smoothness and symmetry of her walking. Then it loosens up more and gets even better when she goes for a walk after her treatment. Esther can immediately tell how much better it looks and feels, delighting in the improvement.

Beware of "Nothing can be done to help you"

Esther's rich, eighty-year life provided her body with ample opportunity to show some wear and tear in a few areas. Looking at aging as a process that can be altered by your actions shows that early intervention and maintaining optimal body function can have enormous effects on the quality of your life.

Twelve months after she first saw me and we began working on her health, Esther is able to move more easily and with much less pain. When she and I review her progress, she expresses gratitude for being so much improved. She was also quite perturbed that her other doctors had all told her that nothing could be done to help her. Out of frustration and concern for others, she asked bluntly, "Why do they do that?"

I didn't have a good answer for as to why, but I told her that "There's nothing to be done" is an answer that is often given to people with chronic health problems. Many of my patients have been told that nothing could be done to help them. Fortunately, they didn't believe their doctors or at least didn't give up.

If those doctors were more conscious of the power of words, they might say it differently, using words to the effect of "There is nothing *I* can do to help you" or "There is nothing that *I* know of that could help you." Both of these convey a different meaning than "There is nothing that can be done to help you." Esther's doctors may have really meant that nothing could be done to help that deteriorated spine on the X-ray, but they were not considering the dynamic, living spine inside this unique person.

Of course, I have not been able to help every patient, and this is sometimes difficult, especially when a patient has been to many other doctors and is seeing me as a last resort. I may tell someone that I can't help and that I may not know who or what could help, but I don't tell patients that nothing can be done to help them. For chronic problems, there is always something you can do to improve your body's function.

Summary of Key Points

Regardless of any disease you may have, acute or chronic, explore ways to improve your health:

1. For any ongoing process of deterioration, consider three valuable possibilities:
   a. Can the process be slowed?
   b. Can the process be stopped?
   c. Can the process be reversed?

2. The human body loves motion, but the parts have to be working properly to fully receive the benefits.

3. A critical factor in maintaining the health of spinal discs is the freedom of motion of the vertebrae above and below each disc. One of the greatest accomplishments of periodic chiropractic treatment is the elimination of spinal fixations and vertebral misalignments, which otherwise cause premature degeneration of the discs.

4. Healthy aging is a process dependent on maintaining normal function of the body.

5. It is not just "You are what you eat." It is "You are what you absorb."

6. Strive to have all three sides of the triad of health—structural, chemical, and emotional—working together on your behalf.

Holistic Healthcare for Health and Fitness

Treating a sports injury and improving athletic performance by looking at health and fitness together

Ellen has always been fit. But she has not always been healthy. As an elite runner, her life has been a series of high-demand performances.

She won many races, held an American running record for a time, and participated in several Olympic trials. Now, at forty-five years old, she is a mother of three and a practicing attorney, and she remains a dedicated runner. She first saw me when a foot problem severely limited her ability to run. The previous year she had fractured a bone in her right foot. Though the fracture healed, the foot wasn't functioning properly, and running further traumatized it.

About five months after she began treatment, during which time she saw me two to four times per month, she reported that her foot had been fine for some time. She had thoroughly tested it by running three full marathons in a period of five weeks, finishing each in less than three hours, with no foot problem. I had not recommended she run three marathons so close together. She chose to, based on her goals, and was able to do so and remain healthy, a testament to her stamina, fitness, and health.

What is significant is that Ellen had not always been healthy. In her twenties and thirties, like many elite athletes, she held certain beliefs that fats were bad. For years, she also struggled with an eating disorder that compromised her nutritional status. Gradually, as we worked together, the functional testing I did with her showed her the specific effects and improved body function from nutrients she had previously been deficient in. She listened and learned with an open mind, and it is a credit to her courage and openness that she now allows herself to consume more healthy proteins and good fats. Even though she is concerned about weighing a few pounds more than she ever has, she recognizes that the health and endurance benefits outweigh her previous beliefs.

Ellen is a great example of how, by actively caring for your body, you can increase your fitness *and* your health. Fitness and health are not the same. People frequently sacrifice their health in order to become more fit. Inevitably, they end up injuring themselves. Too often, they then abandon exercise and join the ranks of wounded warriors destined to become couch potatoes.

While Ellen came to see me only because of her foot problem, correcting it required that together she and I address her overall health and fitness. I wasn't treating a foot problem; I was treating a person with a foot problem. If I had just treated her foot, without considering the rest of her, I probably would not have been able to correct it because only part of the foot problem was located in the foot. She had a misaligned bone and two ankle muscles that were inhibited, or "turned off." Her ankle muscles were not supporting her foot properly, which resulted in the misaligned bone that caused her pain.

But the malfunctioning ankle muscles were innocent bystanders. Nothing was wrong with them; they were just being shut off by problems elsewhere in her body. The light bulb was OK, but the switch was off. Ellen's ankle muscles were inhibited due to misalignments of her pelvis and lower spine as well as an imbalance in her aerobic and anaerobic systems.

Using Applied Kinesiology procedures, I first tested her ankle muscles and then determined what was turning them off. Remember, muscles move bones, so correcting the mechanical problems in her foot required the restoration of normal function to the muscles that support the foot. Her ankle muscles were being inhibited by misalignments in her spine and pelvis, which affected the nerves going to those muscles, so I made mechanical adjustments to correct her spine and pelvis. Now her ankle muscles were able to do their work—to move her foot bones properly and without pain.

Close your medicine cabinet and tap your Inner Pharmacy

Now let's look at how Ellen's muscles were also affected by her Inner Pharmacy and its relationship to her aerobic and anaerobic metabolism. The aerobic system breaks down and burns fats, thereby producing energy. In the course of turning fats into energy, it also produces anti-inflammatory chemicals called prostaglandins. Much more energy is produced from the breakdown of fats than from carbohydrates (sugars). Since fat metabolism produces more sustained energy, it is the foundation for endurance—whether you are running or maintaining your daily health.

But carbohydrates, the staple of the American diet, are not an appropriate foundation for endurance. Carbohydrate metabolism, the basis of the anaerobic system, is more efficient for short bursts of activity. It is what our ancestors used in order to escape from those saber-toothed tigers. But that system wasn't designed for sustained activity, and our ancestors didn't have to constantly run away from tigers. Attempting to use the carbohydrate metabolism for endurance is not only inefficient, but it also becomes highly stressful for the body. The more sugar that is burned as fuel, the more the body has to maintain blood-sugar levels by either eating sugar constantly or by converting stored sugars, proteins, and fats into useable sugar. As the sugar in the blood goes into the muscles to fuel their energy production, the level of sugar in the blood naturally decreases.

To maintain a steady supply of sugar in the blood, the adrenal glands produce a glucocorticoid called cortisol. But cortisol, as it raises the level of blood sugar to support anaerobic activity, becomes a real problem when produced too frequently or in excess. As a stress hormone, if it is produced in excess, it results in high blood pressure, anxiety, insomnia, and a host of other physical maladies. The body then requires more of other nutrients to break down the excess cortisol it is producing.

The quick burst of activity to escape the saber-toothed tiger is different from running for several hours. You can survive running a few hours on adrenaline and cortisol, but at what expense? You deplete the adrenal glands and your body's mechanisms for converting stored sugars, proteins, and fats into immediately useable sugar.

Carbohydrates (sugars) and the sugar-burning anaerobic system are simply not the most efficient way to fuel the body for an endurance event. And I'm not referring to just marathon running. *Healthy aging is ultimately an endurance event.* The same principles that allow you to run a marathon without breaking down apply to your ability to live to perhaps a hundred years of age with a good quality of life.

It is ironic that so many people now take expensive medications to lower their blood-fat levels and anti-inflammatory drugs such as NSAIDs to control inflammation when our own Inner Pharmacies could be doing the same thing efficiently, without expense, drug interactions, or side effects. All we need is to give our bodies the right raw materials and the right kind of exercise that enables our bodies to convert the raw materials into energy and good chemicals.

Let's look at the raw materials, since a dietary imbalance of these is a common cause of aerobic deficiency. First, many people don't consume enough of the good fats necessary to fuel the aerobic system. "Good fats" are naturally occurring fats and oils from plants and fish. They do not include vegetable fats that have been processed. Some animal fats can be considered as good fats as well, but ultimately the issue is one of balance. You want your consumption of good fats to far exceed your bad fats so your body favors the production of good anti-inflammatory chemicals over production of "not-so-good" pro-inflammatory chemicals. Like many athletes and people on "low-fat" diets, Ellen did not consume enough good fats, believing that fats are inherently bad.

The second common imbalance in our diet is the consumption of bad fats, in the form of trans fats or hydrogenated fats and oils. These artificially processed, man-made fats create inflammation and numerous problems in the body and even interfere with your body's ability to metabolize good fats. They should be avoided as much as possible. Trans fats are in fried foods and most processed or packaged foods. The typical Western diet contains far too many trans fats, and this may be one reason why the United States leads the world in the incidence of many degenerative diseases.

The third common dietary imbalance that can cause an aerobic deficiency is consumption of excess carbohydrates, such as refined sugar and white flour and even starches like potatoes. Excess carbohydrate intake and subsequent elevated levels of insulin block the metabolism of good fats. Increased insulin levels can contribute to premature aging and are also implicated in a number of degenerative diseases. Ongoing high-carbohydrate diets require the body to produce excessive amounts of insulin. After years of producing high amounts of insulin, the pancreas can become sluggish and just wear out. The average American consumes over 150 pounds of sugar each year, compared to ten pounds just a century ago.[10] This means the average twenty-year-old has consumed and processed over three thousand pounds of sugar compared to two hundred pounds for a twenty-year-old a few generations ago. Is it any wonder that many people experience problems with their blood-sugar regulation mechanisms?

When we ask our body parts to do a lifetime of work in only ten or twenty years, they simply wear out prematurely.

If you have to produce fifteen times the amount of insulin that your ancestors did, you're going to need at least fifteen times the amount of ingredients and cofactors (such as zinc, chromium, and several of the B vitamins) necessary to produce it. And if your pancreas doesn't have enough raw materials that it needs in order to produce this excessive amount of insulin, it loses its ability to regulate blood-sugar levels and to get sugar into your tissues for fuel. The result is diabetes.

Even the name "adult onset diabetes" has become obsolete because acquired diabetes now occurs frequently in teenagers and children. As opposed to juvenile diabetes (which people are born with), this increase is avoidable. By simply modifying diet and exercise and taking nutritional supplements, the onset of diabetes can be prevented or deferred for many. One of the few things most health experts agree upon is that the less the need for insulin production, the better. Therefore, it is critical to reduce your intake of excess carbohydrates.

Your diet becomes your health. It is your responsibility. Look toward to the future: If people will consume more of the foods "that God made" and less of the foods "that man made," we will be headed in a healthy direction. There is an inherent balance in nature, and artificial trans fats and highly processed, concentrated sugars do not exist there.

To summarize, all of us are at risk for aerobic deficiency from an imbalance in the raw materials and/or not having the right kind of exercise to convert those raw materials into good chemicals. And the common dietary problems that affect the raw materials are (1) not enough good fats, (2) too many bad fats, and (3) too many carbohydrates, or any combination of these three.

It's rather simple. Yet, unless you are somewhat disciplined about your diet, it is easy to screw up on all three of the above, because that is how most people eat, at least in the Western world. It's also why, in addition to maintaining a good diet, my patients supplement their diets with nutrients such as fish oil, flax seed oil, wheat germ oil, black currant seed oil, or sesame oil. This is individualized according to body type, diet, and activity level, but most patients take at least one of these essential fatty acid products as a supplement. (This is discussed further in part 3.)

The other key to correcting the aerobic deficiency is getting your body to convert good fats into good chemicals and energy. The best way to do this is through aerobic exercise, which literally trains the body to burn fat. When done properly, it makes the body burn more fat all the time, not just when you are exercising. You could exercise just thirty minutes a day, and your body will burn more fat in the other twenty-three and a half hours because of what you did and how you did it.

"Aerobic" doesn't just refer to a certain kind of exercise class held at the local health club. Almost any exercise could be made more anaerobic (sugar-burning) or more aerobic (fat-burning). To maximize the aerobic component of your exercise, whatever you choose to do, the most important factor is to elevate and sustain your heart rate. (A formula for determining your appropriate heart rate follows later in this chapter.)

If you exercise at too low or too high a heart rate, you miss out on the benefits from exercise, or worse, you can injure yourself. The most common problem that people develop by exercising improperly is an *anaerobic excess*, which results from exercising at too high of a heart rate.

With an excess of anaerobic activity, your liver often can't keep up with converting enough stored sugar, protein, and fat into useable blood-sugar. Your liver also has to work overtime and use additional nutrients to break down the by-products of the increased anaerobic metabolism, especially lactic acid. When this happens, you typically have more soreness in muscles and joints and may even experience sleep problems, such as waking during the night, due to excess levels of lactic acid. You are also more prone to injury such as sprains or strains.

Even though you can feel great during exercise, because of the high from adrenal hormones, your adrenal glands are, in fact, getting depleted. This "adrenaline rush" is one more chase by the "saber-toothed tiger," one more stressful event for your body. Eventually, fatigued adrenals make it even more difficult to maintain adequate blood-sugar levels during and after exercise, which creates more fatigue and a predisposition for low blood sugar. The subsequent sugar cravings often reinforce the cycle and cancel any benefits from the exercise.

You could have either an aerobic deficiency or an anaerobic excess or both. Aerobic deficiency is common among all people, whether they exercise regularly or not. It is especially common among people who don't exercise, because their Inner Pharmacies don't get the opportunity to convert good fats into energy. It also occurs among people who do exercise, if they are not providing their body with enough "good fats."

Anaerobic excess is quite common among people who exercise regularly but who do most of their exercise at too high of a heart rate and among those who do not warm up or cool down sufficiently.

Ellen had both aerobic deficiency and anaerobic excess when I first tested her. To correct the imbalance, we made some adjustments in her diet, her supplements, and even her training, by slightly lowering her heart rate to minimize the anaerobic stress and maximize her aerobic performance. How I determined that she had aerobic deficiency and anaerobic excess is covered below.

How to know if you have an aerobic deficiency or anaerobic excess

Specific muscle testing, used in functional neurology and Applied Kinesiology, is the most useful diagnostic tool for identifying an aerobic deficiency or anaerobic excess.

The testing is similar to the traditional neurological evaluation of a patient, such as when muscles are tested to look for patterns of weakness, which then can be traced to problems in specific areas of the brain.

With anaerobic excess, you exhibit multiple muscle weaknesses if you place your body under anaerobic conditions. In my office, I have the person run in place or on a treadmill. I then monitor the heart rate, asking them to run until the rate rises to the level I suspect as being anaerobic. If the anaerobic system is working properly, the person's muscles will not become inhibited just because their heart rate is above their ideal aerobic range. Yet with anaerobic excess, many muscles will test weak at higher heart rates because the anaerobic system is being challenged. The muscles themselves are not at fault; they are simply inhibited by malfunctioning physiology. Muscle inhibition causes a greater tendency for injuries, because the muscles are not properly supporting the joints.

Another way to challenge the anaerobic system is to have the patient do rapid muscle contractions, such as flexing and extending their elbows as fast as possible for about ten seconds. People with anaerobic excess will exhibit a temporary weakening/inhibition of many muscles easily identified through manual muscle testing. Within ten or fifteen seconds, the body returns to normal, because the person was in an anaerobic state for a short time. If the anaerobic activity is sustained, the muscle inhibition would continue.

The muscle weakness pattern exhibited in aerobic deficiency is even more interesting and common, because it occurs in many of us, whether we exercise or not. If you test a normal muscle that is facilitated or "on" and test it repeatedly, it will dramatically weaken by the third or fourth test. With aerobic deficiency, normal muscles weaken when they are used repeatedly. Can you see how this would contribute to fatigue and also predispose someone to injury while the muscles are inhibited?

These muscle-testing procedures evaluate for patterns of selective muscle inhibition that occur during specific activities, such as continued running at too high a heart rate or with an aerobic system that has insufficient fuel.

Let's apply this to Ellen's ankle-stabilizing muscles and her ongoing foot problem. Two ankle muscles were inhibited, leaving her foot unsupported. I was able to get those muscles turned on by correcting misalignments in her pelvis and spine. The misalignments created weakness by affecting the nerve supply to those muscles. Once the muscles were functioning normally, I tested them specifically with the aerobic and anaerobic challenges. When I tested them repeatedly, they weakened dramatically, indicating aerobic deficiency. To correct the problem, Ellen added a bit more good fat to her diet and started taking fish-oil capsules.

The muscles also weakened following the anaerobic challenge, which meant that they were not supporting her if she ran at a heart rate higher than her aerobic range. Correcting the anaerobic excess required improving her liver function. She reduced her consumption of sugar (which was not excessive) and artificial sweeteners, which the liver has to break down. We added a nutritional supplement to increase her consumption of B vitamins, especially thiamine or vitamin B1, which the liver uses to break down lactic acid. Ellen's increased amounts of lactic acid from her anaerobic excess required greater amounts of thiamine to metabolize it properly. So she reevaluated her running heart rate and lowered it to maximize the use of her aerobic system and to minimize any further stress on her anaerobic system.

Restoring normal functions to each system, the aerobic and anaerobic, and restoring balance between the two resulted in her ankle muscles staying on properly, even during those three full marathons that she ran. The chiropractic adjustments to her pelvis, lower spine, and foot, along with the Applied Kinesiology corrections to her ankle muscles, were equally effective in allowing her body to function normally.

How to find your optimal exercise heart rate

Several approaches exist for calculating your optimal exercise heart rate. I use a formula developed by a colleague, Dr. Phil Maffetone.[11] He has trained and treated many outstanding endurance athletes over the past thirty years and has learned what does and doesn't work. Like I do, he uses only natural healthcare methods, not drugs or surgery.

Dr. Maffetone's heart-rate formula puts most people at a lower rate than the traditional formula used in athletic training and in most health clubs. Over twenty years of practice, I have found it to be safe and effective at improving both health *and* fitness.

To find your ideal aerobic range, subtract your age from 180. The result is the top number of a range of ten, which is your individual range of optimal heartbeats per minute during exercise. For example, Ellen, at forty-five years old, should have 125 to 135 beats per minute

(180 − 45 = 135). This range can be increased or decreased by five to ten, based on your health, recent injury, current exercise, and whether you take regular medication, as discussed on page 205.

Because Ellen is very fit and attuned to her body, her optimal aerobic rate is about 135 beats per minute. Needless to say, she can run at a higher rate for short bursts, but a higher rate for long periods will put her into an anaerobic excess, sacrifice her endurance, and possibly increase the chance of injury.

The more you develop your aerobic base, the more efficiently your cardiovascular system and fat-burning mechanisms work, the more energy and anti-inflammatory chemicals your body produces from fat, and the greater your endurance becomes with a decreased chance of injury. The aerobic base is like a pyramid. The base and lower half to two-thirds of the pyramid represent aerobic activity, the foundation of the whole physiology that promotes fat-burning, endurance, and healthy aging. The top part of the pyramid represents anaerobic activity, the physiology of sugar/carbohydrate burning, quick-acting activities that are necessary and good but which can become harmful if there is not an aerobic foundation beneath them.

Health *and* fitness come from a balance of aerobic and anaerobic activities, with both systems working efficiently. Each system requires specific nutrients to use as fuel and specific vitamins to assist the conversion of the fuel into energy. The activity of each system is stimulated by exercise at various heart rates.

Unfortunately, there is an epidemic of aerobic deficiency and less so of anaerobic excess. Both are because we are not exercising right, or our diets fail to provide us with necessary ingredients. The result is that many of us give up on exercise far too early in life. And by becoming more sedentary, we tremendously accelerate the aging process. Your body thrives on motion and activity.

I described how I treated Ellen for her foot problem. Another person, complaining of the same pain, might receive significantly different treatment procedures. The common denominator is restoring normal function to the foot. As a holistic practitioner, I treated Ellen, not just her foot. Her foot had been evaluated and treated by sports-medicine doctors and foot specialists—with no results. It got no better until her body got better. That required treating the person: her muscles, her spine, her diet and supplements, her lifestyle.

Diagnosis is more than giving it a name

When Ellen first came to see me, she was concerned with wanting a specific name for her foot problem. It was as though she and I spoke two different languages: she wanted a name for it, especially because every doctor she had seen told her something different. Was it a tendonitis or a plantar fasciitis or perhaps something else? I, on the other hand, was more concerned with trying to figure out what was causing the inflammation and what we could correct to reduce it. She felt relieved when I called it tendonitis. Later, Ellen came to understand why the specific name had held so little significance for me. She understood that her foot was inflamed because of misaligned bones, irritated nerves and muscles that weren't supporting it due to problems in her spine, and an imbalance in her aerobic and anaerobic systems. The foot, as I said earlier, was an innocent bystander to problems elsewhere in her body.

As her body recovered, Ellen was truly amazed at the existence of this holistic approach to healthcare and human performance. It brought her a whole new understanding and appreciation of how nature heals and how the body can heal itself, if you can just get it working properly. She was deeply grateful that she could run again and experience more joy in running than ever before.

It wasn't just Ellen's foot that got better through the treatment. The health of her whole body improved, and her new health and fitness contributed to athletic performance she never expected. That's why I call it *healthcare*. I work with each person to get them healthier, and in the process, many different symptoms simply take care of themselves. Ellen was an ideal patient. She had a healthy degree of skepticism, but nevertheless she followed my recommendations and made the appropriate changes in her lifestyle. She worked *with* me, which is what the doctor-patient relationship should be all about. She engaged in the process, and we worked as a team to get her body functioning better so that her foot could heal and her health could improve. Yes, that is holistic healthcare.

Summary of Key Points

1. It is not necessary to sacrifice your health to increase your fitness.

2. Healthy aging is an endurance event. Work to improve both health and fitness.

3. If your attempts to increase fitness have resulted in injury or illness, reevaluate your exercise and lifestyle strategy.

4. The epidemic of aerobic deficiency is due to
   a. an imbalance in the raw materials you provide to your body, such as
      (1) not enough good fats
      (2) too many bad fat
      (3) too many carbohydrates
   b. not having the right kind of exercise to convert those raw materials into good chemicals.

5. Your heart rate, during exercise, determines the relative amounts of fat or sugar that your body burns as fuel.

6. Exercising at a specific heart rate range can cause your body to burn more fat and proportionately less sugar.

7. Exercising at too high of a heart rate can produce anaerobic excess, resulting in many potential symptoms and an increased chance of injury.

8. Specific patterns of selective muscle inhibition during exercise can be identified and corrected through Applied Kinesiology.

9. Holistic healthcare, which works to normalize body function, can increase health, fitness, and human performance.

Explore and Discover What Could Be Triggering Your Symptoms

The cause of a conductor's shoulder problem was not so obvious

John is a gifted and truly outstanding orchestra conductor. His demanding schedule takes him all over the world to teach, conduct, and arrange music. The tale of his shoulder problem conveys valuable lessons to look beyond a symptom.

John first visited me in 1991 on the recommendation of a friend. His right shoulder had been in constant pain for years, and his internist had progressed from recommending pain relievers to suggesting surgery, a surgery that John, as a layperson, understood as "scraping his tendons." He wanted to avoid surgery if there was any way to improve his shoulder without it. As the son of a physician, he was skeptical about my holistic, alternative approach. But with nothing to lose, he was willing to give it a try, since he felt that if it didn't help, he would need surgery anyway.

During that first consultation, John told me about how some of the greatest conductors mature artistically in their sixties, seventies, and eighties. Ironically, for many, by the time they fully matured in their art, their shoulders were often damaged, worn out, and limited in their range of motion, ravaged by the many years of conducting.

John, then in his mid-forties and frequently conducting eight to ten hours a day, told me that one of his goals was to be able to conduct with large, free, dramatic shoulder and arm motions when he is in his seventies and eighties. When a patient tells me of a health or performance goal, it becomes my goal to help him attain it. I was moved by the beauty of John's goal and committed myself to try to find what was causing his shoulder problem. The issue was not so much to get rid of his current shoulder pain as to help his shoulder work better for the lifetime of conducting that lay ahead.

Other doctors assumed that John's shoulder problem was simply the result of overuse from hours of daily conducting. Their solution was to periodically "take out the garbage," or scrape away the calcium deposits that had piled up from the damage. I looked at it differently. I wanted to figure out how to keep the damage from occurring in the first place.

I knew that if John's shoulder was working properly, it wouldn't become damaged and painful, even with conducting up to ten hours a day. So the question and mission became what to do to improve the function of the shoulder, or in other words, to determine what was preventing the shoulder from functioning in an optimal way. Of course, that meant looking at the person with the shoulder problem, not just at the shoulder.

During the course of analyzing and testing John's whole body, I identified one specific right shoulder muscle that tested as if it was weak or being inhibited. Needless to say, it was not weak due to a lack of exercise, yet it tested just as if it was very weak. The muscle was being turned off by some malfunction in his body. At that point, I felt like I was "hot on the trail," because it was logical that this inhibited muscle was the source of the problem. A couch potato might get by without the support of this shoulder muscle, but not a world-class conductor. Conducting hours a day requires all shoulder muscles to be on, providing support to the shoulder at all times. Instability from this muscle not being on was probably the biggest factor in the chronic inflammation and pain John was experiencing.

In Applied Kinesiology, there is a systematic way to determine what is causing a muscle to be turned off, or inhibited, when it shouldn't be. It requires testing different factors such as the nerve and blood supply to the muscle, lymphatic drainage from the muscle, and specific acupuncture circuits, and then observing which make a difference in the inhibited muscle. In John's case, his inhibited shoulder muscle only tested normal when he held his breath a certain way, which indicated a problem with his cranial bones. Providing additional data for me was the fact that this particular cranial fault was a pattern usually associated with allergies.

I decided to do the simplest thing first: perform the cranial correction by applying gentle pressure on specific cranial bones as he breathed a certain way. This correction to restore normal motion to the bones of his skull took about a minute to perform and immediately reset his body so the shoulder muscle was then on. I also did several other cranial, spinal, and pelvic corrections commonly associated with the specific cranial problem that had been inhibiting his shoulder muscle.

Sometimes the "resetting" of a muscle has an immediate and permanent effect, but more commonly, several corrections are required to maintain the reset. Some of the cranial faults act like "circuit breakers" in the body and can be overloaded by chemical, physical, and even emotional imbalances. Since I suspected that the cranial fault inhibiting John's shoulder muscle was related to allergies, I told him it was possible it could go off again, re-weakening his shoulder. Eating some food that he was allergic or sensitive to would likely be the trigger which would throw it off again.

He looked at me as if I were from outer space. But since his shoulder felt better, he agreed to give it a few days and then be tested again to see if the cranial correction had held and his shoulder muscle had stayed on. I was confident that once the shoulder muscle stayed on permanently, his shoulder would function better and would likely heal on its own.

John returned a few days later with his shoulder somewhat improved, which was a good sign, but I wasn't convinced it was fully corrected yet. Testing revealed that the same muscle was turned off. With further testing, this weak muscle was again strengthened by the same cranial pattern I had corrected earlier. Rather than simply correcting it again, I felt that it was important to address what was likely throwing it off, or "breaking the circuit."

What had happened to John since I last saw him that again overloaded the circuit? Since his pattern of breathing indicated a food allergy, I reviewed John's diet with him. I was not concerned that he may have had a classic allergic reaction to some particular food. But there are "food sensitivities," a type of allergic reaction wherein your body reacts to a food because it may not be able to digest or metabolize it well, or may be getting too much of that food, or perhaps getting it too frequently. Food sensitivities sometimes produce a runny nose, itching eyes, and typical allergic rhinitis symptoms, which can alert people to the allergic nature of the body's reaction. Food sensitivities are also notorious for triggering joint problems. However, when an allergen produces headaches, fatigue, or stiff and painful joints in the hands, feet, knees, and shoulders, people typically don't associate such pains with food, especially because there is often a delay of hours or even days before symptoms appear. It requires detective work to identify the culprits.

There are two rules of thumb for food allergies and sensitivities. One is that we commonly crave the foods we are sensitive to. The other is that we often consume the offending food frequently—sometimes daily or several times a day. John had, overall, a healthful diet. He was not eating a lot of sugar or bad fats. He ate moderate amounts of fruit, vegetables, and protein. What made me suspicious was that he ate wheat at almost every meal: a bagel for breakfast, bread at lunch, and pasta at dinner. He wasn't craving wheat products, but they were his "comfort" foods, and he ate them at least three times a day.

To get more data, I corrected the cranial fault as I had done on the previous visit, which again resulted in an immediate facilitation or strengthening of his problematic shoulder muscle. I then placed a small amount of wheat flour on his tongue. Once he could taste it, I retested the shoulder muscle. Not only did the muscle now test weak, but merely contracting the muscle to do the manual muscle test brought on shoulder pain.

His jaw dropped open and his eyes widened as he looked at me in dismay. He couldn't believe that wheat could immediately affect his body so profoundly. In his own words, he was blown away by his shoulder's reaction to the wheat on his tongue. Just doing the test made it hurt in a way he had not felt for several days. As strange as this seemed to John, his experience was dramatic, and even as a skeptic, he became convinced there was something to it.

I explained that this was a neurological test; the wheat stimulated nerve receptors on his tongue, which send a message directly to the area of the brain that senses tastes. His brain was shutting that muscle "off" in response to the wheat, which it perceived as an offending substance. I emphasized that this was how his body reacted to wheat every time he put it in his mouth!

I recommended that he stop eating anything with wheat in it. His wife suggested he had nothing to lose, and she and his colleagues helped him to live without wheat. Within two weeks, the pain in John's shoulder had totally disappeared. He still had a hard time believing it was wheat-related, but he continued to avoid wheat products. I monitored him, periodically, to see if he could eventually eat wheat in moderation. But each time I tested the wheat on his tongue, the shoulder muscle weakened and I would repeat the cranial correction to reset his body. The following year, when his shoulder pain returned after he accidentally drank wheat beer in Japan, even his most doubting colleagues became convinced of wheat's effect on John's shoulder.

At the time, I didn't know if John had an inherent allergy to wheat, meaning he would probably always react to it, or if his sensitivity came from too much wheat or eating it too frequently, thereby overloading his body's ability to process it. If it were the latter, John could eventually return to consuming wheat in small amounts and infrequently.

After three years, he was able to eat pasta without upsetting his shoulder, as long as he ate wheat only every few days, which reveals that John is not totally allergic to wheat but sensitive to it. His shoulder became a barometer for his wheat sensitivity.

Since 1991, John has had no shoulder pain and never needed shoulder surgery. Furthermore, his overall health has improved. The treatments he received to help his shoulder helped his whole body. What I did was to correct and reset his body so it could heal itself. Even more important, and what may have been the most significant contribution to John's health and well-being, was the detective work brought to John by a holistic approach in which the goal was to determine what wasn't working properly in his body and why. The surprising answer: a shoulder muscle that did not turn on properly due to a food sensitivity.

What might have happened to John had he gone ahead with the shoulder surgery and never discovered the wheat sensitivity? First, even after surgery, that shoulder muscle would still have been weak due to the wheat response. The proposed surgery to clean up debris around his tendons may have removed some past damage, but it would not have made his shoulder function better. He might have had a difficult time healing and rehabilitating from the surgery without the proper muscle support in his shoulder. Even if it did improve after surgery, the shoulder would have deteriorated as time passed from hours of conducting with the muscle still shut off. So his shoulder may have been worse off or, at the very least, caught in a cycle of repeated surgeries, which may eventually have threatened his conducting career.

It is also possible that John's wheat sensitivity, had it gone undetected, could have created other serious problems in his body, such as affecting other joints or creating health and aging problems that could be avoided simply by changing his diet.

What is significant for anyone with chronic problems is that John had no other symptoms commonly associated with an allergic reaction. His wheat reaction affected a specific muscle and joint without causing other obvious problems in his body. Is John's scenario common? Are food sensitivities something to be considered when looking at chronic structural, mechanical problems such as arthritis or even digestive problems?

The answer is yes. Food sensitivities affect many people in various ways. They don't necessarily affect a shoulder muscle, as John's did. But they do frequently affect one or more joints in the hands, feet, knees, shoulders, hips, or spine. Wheat is not the only culprit. It is common because of the inordinate amounts of wheat we consume and perhaps because our bodies have been fooled by so much refined, rather than whole wheat, flour. While almost any food can trigger a reaction in the body, certain foods more commonly affect joints, such as citrus, vegetables in the nightshade family (especially tomatoes and potatoes), dairy products, corn, and chocolate.

This is not to say that everyone with a painful joint has a food sensitivity. People can have painful joints for many reasons: injury, misalignment of the joint, malfunctioning muscles around the joint, or an acid-base or protein imbalance. Nor is it to say that food sensitivities cause only joint problems. They can cause digestive or immune system problems, asthma, and even mood disorders. "Brain allergies," in which it is the brain that reacts to the offending food, can severely interfere with concentration and mental focus and cause many children and adults to be labeled as having ADHD (attention deficit hyperactivity disorder).[12] Anxiety, brain fog, and even panic attacks are often related to food sensitivities, as are asthma and certain skin problems.

Many of us have bloating and discomfort after a meal because we are eating foods that don't agree with our bodies. Unfortunately, we aren't taught that these symptoms are indicators that something is not working properly. We as individuals are responsible for our own health, and we can look for the cause of own digestive or joint symptoms rather than seek immediate relief from symptoms by medications.

Completely ignoring the cause of your symptom means missing the opportunity to identify what may be causing many other chronic problems. It is like ignoring the flashing warning indicator light in a car. You can put tape over it or remove the flashing light, but the problem that triggered it is still there and will likely emerge at some point, possibly as a more severe problem than it was when the light first started flashing.

If a food is triggering an inflammatory reaction in one part of your body, it's likely that increased inflammation is also resulting in other parts. Since inflammation plays a key role in heart disease, there is great value in discovering and eliminating anything that triggers your Inner Pharmacy to produce more bad chemicals and not enough good ones.

With food sensitivities, resulting problems usually become chronic as long as the offending food is consumed regularly. If you have any chronic problem, first consider that your body is always trying to correct itself. The existence of a chronic problem means that something is preventing your body from correcting itself. That something could be a structural, chemical, or emotional imbalance, or any combination of these, and it is happening to your body on a regular, perhaps daily, basis. In John's case, it was primarily chemical. Whatever it is, your goal is to identify and eliminate it before a joint or other symptomatic area is so damaged that it has lost the ability to repair itself.

Of course, there is a point at which a deteriorated area of the body can no longer rejuvenate itself and will need to be removed or replaced, or else the person just has to survive without it. Fortunately, Western medicine has made great advancements in the fields of joint replacement and organ transplants. But however you look at it, replacement therapy should always be Plan B. The much easier and less invasive Plan A is to preserve your own joints and organs for as long as possible.

A holistic approach to healthcare lends itself to identifying and correcting malfunctions in your body and to the wear and tear that causes parts of the body to break down prematurely. This is why holistic care is a good choice if you have a chronic problem, one in which traditional medicine may not even recognize that a problem exists until a certain level of deterioration has already occurred. You don't have to wait until it is time for a joint replacement to do something about excessive wear and tear on your joints. Surgery or not, it is still critical to restore normal function to any body part that is dysfunctional. That's why it is good to see a holistic practitioner and have an evaluation for normal function even if you plan to have surgery. Sometimes you can restore normal function so the area can heal on its own. But if surgery is still necessary, whatever was done to help restore normal function will be helpful in post-surgical healing and rehabilitation. It may even increase the chances of a successful surgery. So, if at all possible, *fix it first*.

Where do food sensitivities come from?

Since food sensitivities are an increasingly common cause of chronic symptoms, let's explore their origin. Are they acquired or innate? In other words, did John develop sensitivity to wheat as an adult? Or did he have it all his life and it started creating problems for him in his forties?

It appears that sensitivities result from a combination of your genetic and biochemical individuality as well as how the imbalanced diets of today don't match the real needs of our bodies. John's body may have tolerated wheat for a lifetime with no problem if he had consumed it less frequently and in smaller amounts. Or if he had been consuming whole wheat versus white flour, in which significant ingredients are removed from the whole wheat during processing, his body may have been able to digest it without depleting something else in the process.

The body uses up various vitamins and nutrients in the course of digesting and utilizing various foods. Digestion of refined flour, for example, depletes zinc and several of the B vitamins. If you continually consume large amounts of a food, drawing from the body's supply of nutrients to digest it without replenishing the nutrients, eventually some part of your body breaks down, either because the mechanism wears out or because there simply aren't enough raw materials necessary to continue the process.

Think of a food you really like, even if it is a sweet like chocolate or ice cream. Now, imagine having it at least three times a day for forty years. You might think that you would never get sick of having it, but *your body might get sick of it*. At some point, your body could lose the ability to digest and assimilate it, particularly if the food is depleting your stores of nutrients that may be needed for other important body functions. Then your body rejects the food and develops a deficiency or a weakness associated with the processing of it, as John's did. It may take five years; it may take sixty years—but eventually an imbalanced diet will catch up with almost anyone.

While I am not an allergist, I treat people who have chronic inflammatory problems that are aggravated by food sensitivities. Inflammation in the body, which often causes joint pain, is often triggered by a reaction to foods. Addressing the food sensitivity can significantly reduce inflammation in the body without anti-inflammatory drugs.

People who eliminate wheat from their diet know how much attention it requires to do so, because wheat is present in so many foods: bread, rolls, muffins, bagels, pasta, pretzels, cereals, cake, and wheat tortillas. Wheat is pervasive. Most of us don't realize how much and how frequently we consume it. And we don't realize that the excess of it can add to the accumulation of stress on our bodies. If you are sensitive to a food, each time you eat it is the chemical equivalent of an attack by the saber-toothed tiger.

The load of accumulated stress builds until your body can no longer take it, and something breaks down. That's the aging process, and inattention to the cause of chronic problems often accelerates it. Ignoring or medicating for common symptoms without investigating the potential causes of the symptoms is missing a great opportunity to improve your health and to prevent serious problems later on.

John's wheat allergy affected his shoulder muscle; others with the same allergy may develop headaches or intestinal upset or advancing heart disease. Whatever the food, it becomes a trigger for an inflammatory reaction; your genes determine what tissues in your body are affected by the increased inflammation.

As you now know, the mainstream medical approach is oriented toward acute illness and treating diseases rather than trying to solve chronic problems. Chronic problems, however, lend themselves to the evaluation of body function. When you see how little mainstream healthcare offered to John, you can understand its limitations. The same is true for Chris, Pete, Richard, Esther, and Ellen. In each case, the medical approach was to consider their condition as a given, as something permanent that they already had. There was no attempt to identify the cause. The diagnosis was limited to naming the condition. Then doctors tried to make the person more comfortable by medicating the symptoms caused by the condition.

A holistic approach, on the other hand, looks at the symptom as part of a process gone wrong. The medical approach to John's shoulder problem did not attempt to determine if something biomechanical wasn't working properly in his shoulder. It simply accepted his shoulder problem as the product of wear and tear. The possibility that it resulted from a food sensitivity was not considered. John's case is not unique. Many joint problems are categorized as arthritis without considering whether something in the person's body or lifestyle could be triggering it.

Beyond standard allergy tests

In the classic allergic reaction, called an IgE type reaction, there can be an immediate and sometimes life-threatening onset of symptoms, even anaphylactic shock in which the air passageways close down.

John's reaction to wheat was most likely what the allergy world calls an IgG type allergic reaction. IgG reactions are not as acute; instead, they often cause delayed symptoms such as joint or muscle pain, headaches, and fatigue, and it sometimes takes twenty-four to forty-eight hours after eating the offending food for them to appear. They usually result from eating too much of a particular food too frequently over a given period of time.

While it is possible to have both IgE and IgG reactions to a food, I doubt that John would have an IgE reaction to wheat, since he was eventually able to return to consuming it with no problem as long as he reduced the frequency and amount. Furthermore, if someone had evaluated him only for IgE reactions to foods, as is commonly done with skin testing, they would have concluded that he had no reaction to wheat.

Would John's wheat sensitivity have been identified through standard allergy tests? The answer is maybe, based on the fact that there are several types of allergy tests, and they sometimes get varying results because they measure different things. I commonly use blood testing to look for possible allergic reactions, and I could have had lab tests done or even referred John to a traditional allergist. But it makes sense to do the simplest things first. By proceeding to treat John based on the data I obtained, both he and his insurance company were spared considerable expense. More significant, he was treated and improved before we would have received the results of laboratory studies. If his shoulder had not improved, however, I would have tested other foods and may have done some laboratory testing. It simply wasn't necessary in his situation.

There are new and progressive methods that are often successful at desensitizing people to foods they had previously reacted to. I use some of these methods but primarily rely on removing the offending food from the diet for a period of time and then reevaluating after several weeks. There is one thing that almost everyone who deals with allergies agrees on: *The bottom line is how the patient does when he or she eliminates the suspected food.* If symptoms improve when the suspected food is eliminated, there is probably a connection.

Don't let your symptoms limit your choice of healthcare

Whether traditional allergy testing would have identified John's wheat sensitivity depends on what tests are done and what is measured. But there is a bigger question that reveals a major deficiency in our medical system: What would have prompted John to consult with an allergist for his shoulder problem in the first place?

He had no way of being directed to an allergist. Our medical system is primarily symptom-based, so he took himself to an orthopedist because he had pain in his shoulder. Symptomatically, it was an orthopedic problem.

John did not know, because of the way our culture has taught us, that his symptom was the result of an underlying functional problem. Like most of us, he let his symptom dictate where he went for help. Then the orthopedist, who specializes in the symptom of shoulder pain, evaluated John's shoulder, found damage, and would have proceeded to clean up some of the damage.

But the orthopedist looked only at John's shoulder, not at John the person. He didn't address potential malfunctions that were causing the damage, and he didn't give much credit to the possibility of the healing power of nature taking care of the shoulder if normal function could be restored.

Of course John didn't take himself to an allergist. That would have required knowing the specific malfunction creating his shoulder pain. It would have also required an open-minded allergist who performed the type of allergy tests that would reveal John's wheat sensitivity and who could then relate it to his shoulder pain.

Remember, almost all symptoms result from underlying dysfunction. That is why it is so important to match the treatment to the patient. The one-size-fits-all approach to treating symptoms, without individualizing diagnosis and treatment to the various underlying dysfunctions, is quite limited. When you have a chronic problem, consider a healthcare provider who is a generalist. By looking at you holistically, he or she can enhance the matching process. Someday, I hope we will have "dysfunction-based protocols" that doctors of all types can agree on and follow. Then we will all do a better job of attaining successful outcomes for specific symptoms and improving the health of our patients through normalizing the function of their bodies and guiding them to more active, healthy lifestyles.

What I did with John and his shoulder problem was not magic or intuitive or some form of exotic healing. It was simply *identifying and correcting faulty physiology*, which then allowed his body to function normally and to heal itself. When that happened, he was free of a painful, annoying, limiting symptom—and free to live his dreams and to achieve his goals.

Being a holistic doctor means being a "people doctor" as opposed to a "parts doctor." Most of my patients appreciate being looked at as people, not as parts. And it's what I love about being a holistic doctor. It's not that I want to deal with food sensitivities, aerobic/anaerobic imbalances, diaphragm weaknesses, and malfunctioning feet that don't properly turn muscles on. But those are all common problems that cause many other chronic symptoms in the body. Out of necessity, I have had to deal with them to improve body function so that people's bodies can heal properly and get well on their own. Healthcare means taking care of health, and health requires attaining and maintaining normal function for as long as possible.

Summary of Key Points

1. For any symptom, consider what possible malfunction could be causing it. Don't just continually medicate the symptom so you can forget about it. Look for the cause and for what could be triggering the symptom.

2. A huge difference exists between (a) just relieving the pain and (b) improving the function of an area.

3. "Overuse" injuries often have an underlying malfunction that accentuates the problem.

4. Inflammation means that the Inner Pharmacy is producing too many pro-inflammatory chemicals and not enough anti-inflammatory chemicals.

5. Food sensitivities are a common trigger for inflammation anywhere in the body.

6. Delayed allergic reactions to foods often cause chronic symptoms.

7. If you have a chronic symptom and are concerned about potential food sensitivities, be suspicious of (a) any food you crave and (b) any food you eat frequently.

8. Different types of allergy tests measure different reactions. Traditional IgE allergy testing, including skin testing for immediate reactions, may not identify the delayed reactions that cause chronic problems.

9. Specialization in traditional medicine is "symptom-based" or "compartment-based" relative to the region of the body that exhibits the symptoms. Specialization in the CAM professions is more "dysfunction-based."

10. Restore and maintain the normal function of your Inner Pharmacy.

5

What Holistic Healthcare Looks Like in Real Life

Earlier chapters told the histories of real patients. Each offered the opportunity to explore aspects of what it means to have a normally functioning body. Each showed that good function can actually be restored and maintained through true healthcare and through giving your body good materials to work with and treating it to a healthy lifestyle.

In this chapter, you'll see what it means to seek healthcare that treats *you* holistically. The three components of your health—structural, chemical, and emotional—are addressed through the story of a hypothetical patient, Tom, who has a knee problem. He is a compilation of frequent patterns and scenarios I have seen hundreds of times, a kind of healthcare "everyman." He is a baby boomer who has pushed himself hard for years. As a physician (as are many of my patients), he provides a healthy dose of skepticism and a contrasting point of view. Most of us can relate to much of his history as well as to the numerous challenges he faced.

Addressing the Structural Component of Health

Tom came to see me hoping I could help his knee, at least enough to reduce his pain and help him to play sports again. He hated being inactive and was concerned that he was out of shape and that his sporting days were over. A traditional medical approach had helped to manage his knee's pain and inflammation. He and his orthopedic doctor anticipated a knee replacement in the future. As a doctor himself, he never looked at his knee problem as something that was potentially correctable. He had been living with it and waiting for the day when it became debilitated enough to require surgery.

I explained that I look at the person with a knee problem, not just at the knee. I also volunteered to explain what I was doing and why, so that he would have a firsthand experience of how I evaluate and treat a problem. I was happy to proceed in this way, because I always want for people to look at their own bodies in a functional way and realize that many health problems are actually modifiable conditions.

As soon as I saw Tom take a few steps, I thought I could help him. He was puzzled at my confidence and asked why I thought I could help his knee problem without even knowing his history or examining him.

I explained that a high percentage of chronic knee problems exist because of malfunctions and are, therefore, functional knee problems. Most likely, his was a functional knee problem, and correcting the malfunctions would very likely improve his knee. I would have felt differently if a ligament been totally torn, if a loose fragment were floating around his knee, or if the cartilage was completely destroyed. But those possibilities were unlikely, given how he stood and walked.

Although he had not yet told me which knee had the problem or given me his history, Tom was amazed when I told him several problems I could see with his left knee, simply by observing him move. I described a pattern I have seen hundreds of times: his pain was probably on the front-medial side (the inner side) of the knee. Further, while the knee is stiff, the pain probably feels better in the morning and worsens throughout the day. Standing and walking probably aggravate it. The pain may be helped by anti-inflammatory medications, but the knee probably feels unstable—as though it could give out if he moved wrong or tried to run. I told him that he had probably had a medial meniscus injury (injury to the cartilage on the inner side of the knee), at least once, and that his X-rays probably show a moderate loss of joint surface over the medial tibial plateau (the inner side of the knee joint).

He jokingly asked if I was a psychic or magician. No, I told him. Each of those observations was easy to conclude from his posture and movements. I could see how his lower back, knee, and ankle were each misaligned in a way that shifted the mechanical stress onto the inside of his knee.

Dr. George Goodheart, a great physician and my teacher for many years, always told us to "see with eyes that see." In other words, holistic practitioners must develop our powers of observation.

Next, I had Tom remove his shoes so he could see how much his left ankle pronated, i.e., the inner arch dropped when he stood. I showed him how his ankle pronation caused the tibia (the lower leg) to rotate inward, creating medial knee instability. I was fairly sure he had sprained his left ankle at some point and that it never healed properly.

He said, yes, he had sprained the left ankle badly playing basket-ball twenty-five years earlier. He was skeptical that an old ankle injury could still be affecting his knee. From my biomechanical and func-tional point of view, it certainly could. The ankle was changing the position of his knee. Furthermore, his ankle probably wasn't absorb-ing shock properly, which meant that all the shock from the impact of walking was going straight up into his knee, particularly the inner side of the knee. I suggested to him that standing and walking on hard sur-faces especially bothered his knee. He said that was true.

I then showed him how his pelvis was not level. The left side was over an inch higher than the right. This type of pelvic misalignment also creates instability of the medial knee.

Looking at his left knee, he could see it had a "knock-kneed" appearance. That position indicated weakness of his inner knee and added mechanical stress to the medial collateral ligament. It also meant that muscles which should normally support the medial knee were not doing their jobs.

The altered biomechanics of Tom's ankle, knee, and pelvis were causing extra wear and tear, as well as premature degeneration of the inner portion of the knee. Once someone has lost the joint surface, the articulating cartilage of the knee, it is gone forever. It makes sense to do what you can to extend the life of your existing cartilage.

I could also tell, by watching him walk, that at least three specific muscles were "shut off" and not supporting his pelvis, knee, and ankle. Knowing the interrelationships of those muscles helped me understand what was causing his body to "shut them off" and what treatment may be needed to restore them to normal function.

Since each of those misalignments and malfunctioning muscles are normally correctable, I told Tom that I should be able to help his knee quite a bit. If I could get it functioning better, the biggest limitation would be the amount of deterioration and loss of joint surface that had taken place over the previous twenty-some years while he had the structural problems and the poor shock absorption. I reserved the right to change my opinion if something unusual surfaced during his history and examination.

In my explanation to Tom, I emphasized *the difference between the symptom itself and the dysfunction causing the symptom.* To a holistic practitioner such as myself, medial knee pain usually exists because of various potential factors that alter the body's biomechanics and increase the stress on the medial knee.

Improving a symptom without drugs or surgery requires altering the mechanisms that are creating the symptom. To you, a great benefit from a holistic approach is that not only does the symptom improve, but your overall body function improves as well. For Tom, making the corrections necessary to improve his knee would also improve the function of his ankle, his lower back, and other parts of his body affected by his spine. And if his knee could be improved enough so that he could return to more physical activity, sports, and exercise, then his cardiovascular system, energy, fitness, bone strength, flexibility, coordination, and emotional well-being would all be helped. Now that's an exciting set of possibilities!

At this point Tom told me he would be happy for me to make whatever corrections I could. He also told me that, as much as he loved playing sports, especially basketball, he hated to exercise. This emphatic comment made me suspicious of a particular emotional factor that could be affecting his health. There are some phenomenal new techniques that can help change such attitudes, so I told him we might want to deal with that later on. For now, the best place to start was to get his whole history and to evaluate his body. I told him to just assume that I knew nothing about him or his knee and to describe his knee problem, starting at the beginning when it first became a problem.

Tom's story

During medical school, Tom was playing basketball, and his knee twisted and gave out. He wasn't hit but was simply changing directions rapidly. He fell hard, but it was the twisting that injured his knee. The medial collateral ligament was sprained but not torn. It had been loose ever since. The meniscus wasn't torn either, so he had never had surgery. The injury was acutely painful, and Tom walked on crutches for about two weeks. Once it calmed down, he did standard rehabilitation exercises for a while. They helped somewhat, but in the twenty years since the injury, his knee had consistently felt weak and vulnerable.

Tom had tried playing basketball a few times after that. He used a knee brace, but he couldn't move fast, and the knee became painful and inflamed easily. He could calm it with medications, but it never felt right. He feared it would give out again and get more torn up. It felt like it could catch or lock. So he hadn't run in twenty years, and he had done no other significant exercise for a long time. He felt flabby and old and admitted that he was not the best model of health for his own patients. His knee was really holding him back.

The pain was primarily on the medial side and worsened as the day progressed—the longer he stood and walked on it. He would often have to sit for a few minutes to take the pressure off of his knee.

I also wanted to know about his overall health, even if it seem unrelated to his knee. He said that he was more fatigued than he thought he should be, and the fatigue was worse if he had not eaten in a few hours. He never felt great. He didn't digest protein well, which gave him frequent gas, bloating, and heartburn. He was taking medication to control his stomach-acid production, which seemed to help the heartburn. But protein still bothered him, so he just avoided it and ate mainly carbohydrates. He was open to any suggestions about his poor digestion, so I mentioned how faulty mechanics of the diaphragm muscle can allow stomach acid up into the esophagus.

When I evaluated him, I told him that I would look at his diaphragm function, something I routinely check because it rarely functions optimally, and improving it helps the body in so many ways. A dysfunctional diaphragm commonly contributes to fatigue as well as digestive problems.

I asked if he took any other medications besides the antacid.

His reply was, "Just an antidepressant," for the past twenty years or so. He was "down," when he couldn't play sports anymore, because of his knee. He had felt a lot better physically and emotionally when he was active. He said he felt like he was a hundred, and he didn't want to think about what he might feel like in another twenty years. He also said that he frequently took a non-steroidal anti-inflammatory drug (NSAID) for the knee pain and qualified his comment by adding, "if you also count that as a medication."

I replied that of course it is. I was concerned that it could be having serious side effects and asked him to tell me what he meant by "frequently." The answer was almost every day, often a couple of times a day. The NSAIDs sometimes upset his stomach, but he did get a lot less pain and swelling in his knee.

I thought that was a lot, especially if he had been taking that much since the knee injury twenty years earlier. I reserved my NSAID comments for later and continued with his history, asking about surgeries or other major injuries. He told me more about that bad sprain of his left ankle, about twenty-five years ago, a good five years prior to the knee injury. I had guessed right about that from observing the pronation of his left foot. It was a typical inversion sprain, where his foot rolled under him. It was a major sprain, but he didn't think anything had been torn, and it was at least three months before he could run on it. He had turned it a couple of times since then but had had no significant sprains like that first one. He mentioned that it was probably a good thing he was no longer running, at least as far as his ankle was concerned, because he realized that he could have really injured it again if he had stepped wrong.

I asked about recent X-rays or MRIs of his knee. He never had an MRI, but X-rays from last year showed a significant wearing away of the joint surface on the medial side of the tibial plateau, just as I predicted.

I asked about recent blood tests and if there was anything unusual to report from laboratory studies. He was having standard blood tests every few years, and most of the numbers fell in the normal ranges. I wanted specific numbers to evaluate his protein digestion problem and the accelerated deterioration of his knee joint. It is important to use strict and specific criteria for protein levels when considering joint problems. He agreed to get me the numbers.

In his last few blood tests, his triglycerides were quite elevated and much higher than normal. His lack of exercise didn't help, but Tom was puzzled that they would be so high. His cholesterol numbers had always been OK.

Admitting that he did no regular exercise, he said it was like he had a mental block. He knew he could find things to do that wouldn't hurt his knee. The only thing he did regularly was sit-ups and crunches for his abdominal muscles.

I asked if there was anything else that he thought I should know. Since the basic history pretty well covered it, we moved on. Everything so far gave important data about Tom. Now we were going to get additional data—about what was functioning properly in his body and what wasn't. I would describe what I was finding as we went along.

Looking at normal and abnormal

First, I looked at him standing in front of a posturometer grid that allowed me to precisely measure the right-to-left difference in the height of his pelvis, shoulders, and head. His appearance confirmed my earlier observations about his uneven pelvis, genu valgum or "knock-knee," especially on the left, and moderate foot pronation on the left. From the side, his shoulders and upper back appeared quite kyphotic (hunched forward). That position compromises diaphragm function and was probably contributing to his heartburn and fatigue.

His flat abdominals were doing too good of a job of pulling down and forward on his chest. Many athletes have that problem. They overdevelop their abdominals because they like the ripped appearance, yet don't equally develop their back extensor muscles along the whole spine, which help keep the body upright. In addition to pulling down on the rib cage and making a person hunched over, tight abdominals also decrease thoracic excursion, meaning the chest cannot move freely to take in deep breaths. That can compromise oxygen delivery to all parts of the body and reduce performance and endurance. With the body, it's not good to emphasize form over function.

A hunched back is a fairly standard component of the aging process. People lose the tone of their back muscles, and their bones get softer. But why accentuate that posture and age prematurely by exercising your abdominals and nothing else? You don't have to lose the tone of your back muscles. I explained that even though Tom was standing, it's almost like his body still thinks it is sitting.

His sarcastic response was, "That's just great. I do one exercise to try to help, and I'm screwing myself up by doing it."

I certainly didn't want to discourage exercise. But it was extremely important for him to add exercises to tone his back extensor muscles and stretch the abdominals more to deepen his breathing. It would help his diaphragm, his energy, and his digestion. A few simple exercises can accomplish this in minutes per day.

I reassured Tom that his lack of exercise over the past twenty years might not have been so bad, in light of his misaligned left ankle, knee, and pelvis. Frankly, it's likely that weight-bearing exercise would have done more harm than good, like driving a car with no shock absorbers and a badly misaligned front end. He might have further injured his knee and ankle and added unnecessary wear and tear to his hips and spine.

One of my goals was to improve the function of his body so that exercise could again become his ally. Receiving benefits from exercise, without undue wear and tear, requires the body's biomechanics to work properly.

I asked Tom to lie on his back on the examination table. Orthopedic tests to evaluate the knee showed that the medial collateral ligament was quite loose, which usually indicates the medial knee-stabilizing muscles are not doing their jobs. Other ligaments were fine.

Before I checked the actual alignment of his knee, I measured how his feet lined up with him lying on his back, which told me a lot about pelvic alignment and the knees' biomechanics. His left leg lined up about three-quarters of an inch shorter than his right. The left leg was not necessarily shorter; rather, the difference in length was most likely a functional leg-length difference, and is very common, often due to a misalignment in the pelvis. True structural leg-length differences, where the bones are actually a different length, are much less common. In realigning Tom's pelvis, his legs would probably even out and the structural stress on his knee would become more evenly distributed.

He was surprised at the three-quarters of an inch leg-length difference and the potential that they could become even in length by realigning his pelvis. No one had ever looked at his leg length before, and he realized how much that could be affecting his knee. He then asked if the realignment might help his near-constant lower-back pain.

He hadn't mentioned his low-back pain in his history, because he thought it was normal—something everyone has. I explained that it is not normal, especially for people whose lower backs are aligned properly and who have their muscles functioning in a balanced manner.

When Tom stood, his un-level pelvis represents the same misalignment that is giving him a functional short leg on the left when he lies down. Standing, it shifts more weight to the inside of his left knee and also shifts the weight-bearing balance between the left and right hips and left and right ankles. The asymmetry is further complicated by his malfunctioning left ankle. Even the right-to-left balance of the vertebrae and discs in his lower spine are affected. Each of those areas is degenerating prematurely by the excess wear and tear from the misalignment. I asked if that sounded like something we should address.

"Of course," he replied. He hadn't meant to make light of his lower-back pain. He didn't think of it as an indication that his spine and discs, or hips for that matter, could be under excessive wear and tear or that it was a modifiable process. He lived with the pain, at times using pain medication or muscle relaxants.

113

Once Tom had thought about it for a few moments, both as a doctor and as a patient, it made sense that if nerves are continuously irritated and sending pain messages, something isn't right. Ignoring lower-back problems could be accelerating the aging process. He was beginning to understand the larger picture: His knee is related to the rest of his body, and it could never fully heal, partly due to problems in his pelvis and ankle. I was the first doctor to look at *him*, not just his knee. And from that viewpoint, I believed I could improve the function of his damaged knee. But it was going to require improving the function of his whole body.

Since Tom was a doctor, I asked him how often he saw X-rays of elderly people that showed one hip degenerated much more than the other. "Very frequently," he replied.

People who need a hip replacement usually chalk it up to wear and tear or old age. When patients tell me that one hip or knee is worn out from old age, I ask them how old the other side is. They usually get the picture. One side wore out prematurely due to excessive wear and tear or altered biomechanics. I try to promote normal biomechanics earlier in life *before* joints are worn out. I want to do everything possible to extend the life of all parts, and that means taking care of people physically, chemically, and even emotionally.

Correcting Tom's structure

Returning to Tom's leg-length difference, I started working on the misalignments that were affecting his knee. I started with the pelvic misalignment that was pulling up on the left leg, making it shorter than the right. To check the sensitivity of a specific point on the inside of his knee, I pressed on it and asked him to let me know if the point was painful.

He jumped in response to the examining pressure. That point was extremely painful and was an area that usually bothered him when standing or walking. He was familiar with the anatomy of the area but was quite surprised at the localized sensitivity of that specific point.

I explained that this is a point where several muscles which support the inside of the knee attach to the bone. Those muscles, which also pull forward on the same side of the pelvis, had been strained and shut off for a long time. I would be working to reset them so they could support both his pelvis and the inside of his knee.

To begin the corrections, I placed blocks or wedges under his pelvis in specific locations that would help his pelvis realign itself. This is one type of chiropractic adjustment, and gentle as it is, it is quite effective in repositioning the bones. It also affects mechano-receptors in the sacroiliac joints of the lower back such that those nerve endings signal information to the nervous system about the new position of the pelvis.

After about a minute, I removed the blocks from under his pelvis. When I re-measured his legs, they were now even, which confirmed that he did, in fact, have a functional leg-length difference. If the bones of his legs were actually different in length (a structural leg-length difference), they would not have evened out by adjusting his pelvis. When I again pressed on the point on the inside of his knee to see if the pain was reduced, he was astounded that the same point with the same pressure was no longer sensitive. The pain was totally gone, and he naturally questioned whether I was pressing as hard.

Yes, I was using the same pressure. And yes, it is amazing. Our bodies are amazing. The muscles that attach at that point had proba-bly been trying to realign his pelvis for twenty years and were not able to do so because of how they were strained and shut off.

Let's step back for a minute and revisit the thought process. The initial question was whether I could help Tom's knee. His body's response to the pelvic adjustment meant that I could influence his knee pain. The next challenge was to correct the rest of the faulty bio-mechanics and get his body to maintain these corrections.

By correcting bone misalignments and resetting muscles that hold the bones in alignment, the biomechanics improve. Simple. Tom real-ized that if he had known about this kind of holistic healthcare when he first injured his knee, it could have been realigned and reset then. It could have healed properly; he could have been playing basketball all these years; and he might not have a degenerated knee.

Had Tom known to have his ankle bones manually realigned and the muscles reset after his ankle injury, he might have avoided the knee injury that occurred five years later. His knee injury happened because the knee twisted and just gave out, which is often the case. It wasn't that he was hit or had an impact to his knee. For his knee to give out, as he described, it's most likely that one or more muscles were not firing properly. The muscles were shut off and not supporting the knee, so it twisted and gave out. Given his previous ankle sprain, it is very possible that the nerve endings in the ankle joints were not signaling properly to his "knee-supporting" muscles about the need for support. So as he stepped down on his malfunctioning left ankle, the nerve endings, also called mechanoreceptors, didn't signal to his nervous system to turn on the left medial knee muscles.

Another possibility is that his pelvis was already misaligned prior to the knee injury and may have contributed to the knee giving out. Some of the same muscles that support the inside of the knee also support the front of the pelvis. If those muscles were inhibited or shut off by some other malfunction in his body, they may have allowed for the pelvis and lower-back instability as well as the lack of support for the knee. It is possible if some correction had been done to his ankle and maybe his pelvis twenty years ago, he might not have even injured his knee. Knees don't just give out, as his did, when everything is functioning properly. My guess is that he was "an accident waiting to happen."

Sometimes looking back at a series of injuries creates the proverbial chicken-or-the-egg dilemma. Regardless of what was malfunctioning and making Tom vulnerable to a knee injury twenty years ago, it is still potentially correctable.

What would it be worth to Tom to not have had the knee injury in the first place? Or even if he had had the injury, to have his injuries heal properly so that he could have continued the active life he enjoyed? *What is the value of slowing down the aging process?* You can see why I am so passionate about promoting the normal function of the body and working to restore it after an injury. It gives you time and increases your quality of life. It preserves your ability to be active. I want people to join the *longevity revolution* and be able to exercise into old age.

We all have "weak links" in our system—some we were born with and some we acquire through injury or poor lifestyle choices.

Wellness means identifying and strengthening our weak links, not just dealing superficially with the symptoms they create.

In Tom's case, even as a doctor, he treated his own symptoms only with medications, never knowing to investigate the faulty mechanics of his knee. X-rays of his right knee showed no deterioration of the joint surface; the left knee showed significant deterioration. Yet his knees are the same age. What is different is the biomechanics, the function of the two knees. The advanced deterioration of his left knee was the result of faulty biomechanics, poor alignment, muscle instability, and poor shock absorption that he had been living with for twenty years or more.

That deterioration did not stem from one twisting fall, a fall where the knee didn't even receive an impact. Instead, it came from an abnormal structure and function, both of which were correctable.

I was confident that when Tom stood up from the pelvic correction, he would notice that his lower back felt better as well. But I didn't want him to get up yet—not until I did some additional adjustments to lock in that pelvic correction and realign the ankle and the knee itself.

We continued to talk about the difference in healthcare philosophies. He regretted not being more open-minded about exploring options and alternatives for his knee. He said that he realized, almost twenty years ago, that traditional Western medicine didn't have anything to offer to improve his knee. Instead of looking further, he gave up, accepting the knee problem as something that would never get better and would always limit him. That was when he became depressed. He was grateful that at least Western medicine came through and helped him with antidepressant medication.

The next step was to deal with the misalignments of Tom's knee and ankle. It made sense to treat the ankle first, because when he stood, his pronated foot would immediately re-create stress on his medial knee. I began to evaluate the function of the ankle muscles with manual muscle tests of several ankle-supporting muscles. Finding two of them "shut off," I reset the muscles. I then retested them.

Tom shook his head, amazed at how much better the muscles contracted after the corrections, especially when he realized that the muscles could have remained off for the rest of his life, had they not been corrected. Once the ankle muscles were back on, I told him that the corrections would likely have to be done another time or two to be permanent, although often corrections "hold" the first time, even on a very old injury. I gave Tom foot exercises to build the supporting muscles. I also recommended that he get orthotics (customized shoe inserts). They would support his medial arch, counter his pronation, and prevent his knee from rotating inward, where it has been weak for so long. The orthotics wouldn't require special shoes, and I could have them made from a mold of his feet.

Bridging a prejudice bred from unfamiliarity

Tom said that in his medical education, students were told to be wary of chiropractors. He never really knew what was involved with chiropractic. He knew it dealt with misaligned bones and manipulating joints, but he had no idea of the significance of properly aligned bones and joints. When it comes to treating the body to restore normal function, manual adjustments to joints and manipulation to muscles constitute a big part of what chiropractors do. Adjustments are all based on restoring normal function to the body so the body can heal itself. The biggest misconception people have about chiropractic is that it has to do with bones and that chiropractors are bone doctors. It's really much deeper than that.

Traditionally, chiropractors are back or spine doctors and are effective in treating people with structural problems. But chiropractic isn't just for back pain. Because the spine houses the nervous system, which controls body functions, when the function of the spine is improved through chiropractic corrections, many body functions improve as well. Because spinal and cranial problems affect the nervous system, and corrections to these areas improve neurological function, it is more accurate to think of chiropractors as nervous-system doctors.

Tom's pelvic adjustment reduced his knee pain, partly because it affected the nerves to the knee itself and partly because it affected nerves that stimulate muscles around the knee, which then allowed the muscles to alter the biomechanics of his knee. It shows how structure and function are so interconnected. Correcting a structural misalignment in his pelvis not only changed the structure and biomechanics of his knee, but it also affected the nerve supply to his knee-supporting muscles. The improved neuromuscular function helped to sustain the correction when he got up and walked.

Correcting a spinal problem has the potential to stimulate normal function in any part of the body which is influenced by the nerves in that region of the spine. Earlier, I talked about making cranial corrections on several patients. Besides reducing their head pain by improving structural alignment, these adjustments were done in order to stimulate specific nerves and the parasympathetic portion of the autonomic nerve system. The structural adjustment changes the function of the areas that are stimulated by those nerves.

The adjustment to Tom's ankle realigned the bones and immediately improved the *structure* and biomechanics of his ankle, knee, and pelvis. But more important, the adjustment normalized the function of mechanoreceptors in the ligaments of his ankle so they properly stimulated the muscles to "turn on" and support the ankle, knee, and pelvis.

The result of chiropractic adjustments to the spine and joints is improved function of the nervous system, which controls the whole body. Chiropractic is about biomechanical and neurological integrity; it is about health, wellness, human performance, and quality of life.

As are many people, Tom is beginning to understand the existence of a holistic approach that provides many options for one's health. Unfortunately, his knee, spine, and lifestyle took an unnecessary beating before he came to that understanding.

Improving your shock absorption

Next was an Applied Kinesiology test to evaluate whether a weight-bearing joint is absorbing shock properly. I started by testing one of Tom's hip muscles, the left gluteus medius muscle, to make sure it was on. With Tom still lying on his back, I asked him to bring his left leg out about forty-five degrees and to hold that position as I pushed in on his leg. The muscle locked nicely against my examining pressure, and he noticed that it felt quite strong, because it was on and firing properly. Next came the actual test. If the mechanoreceptors and nerve endings in his ankle were working properly, he would pass.

Using my fist, I gently pounded several times on the bottom of his left foot to simulate the activation of nerve endings, as from the impact of walking. If the mechanoreceptors activate properly, the hip muscle stays on. When I retested the gluteus medius muscle, Tom was stunned that he was unable now to hold his leg out against the resistance. Clearly the muscle had shut off, and with a little contemplation, he understood that the impact of my pounding on his foot triggered muscle weakness in his hip—exactly what happens every time he takes a step.

Malfunctioning joint receptors had been signaling the wrong information to his nervous system, shutting off the very muscles they should normally turn on. While it felt and tested very weak after the impact to the foot, there was nothing actually wrong with his gluteus medius muscle. It was simply the "innocent victim, " doing exactly what it is being told to do by his nervous system. Several other lower-back, hip, and knee-supporting muscles were acting the same way with every step Tom took. Over the years, this malfunction caused the deterioration of his left knee and hip. If his left leg took three thousand steps a day over twenty-five years, that's twenty-seven million impacts which weakened his left knee and hip-supporting muscles. Like driving a car over twenty-seven million bumps with no shock absorption, the damage is cumulative.

Many of us have this poor ankle function and don't even know it. We don't think about it because we may not be bothered by ankle pain. We are, however, often bothered by knee, hip, or lower-back pain and sometimes even neck and shoulder pain. Poor ankle function may be to blame if the symptom gets worse later in the day or the longer you are on your feet, or if you have a history of a past ankle injury.

You'll find tremendous value in identifying and correcting such a problem and restoring normal shock-absorption function in the ankle. It not only reduces wear and tear on your body, it promotes normal function. I have made adjustments to many world-class runners and even star NFL football players who had badly injured ankles. One NFL player had already undergone two surgeries to reconstruct and hold together his ankle. Restoring normal alignment, muscle function, and shock absorption of his ankle made a huge difference in his speed and endurance, without his ankle becoming inflamed. After those corrections, he went on to win three Super Bowl rings.

I proceeded to adjust Tom's ankle to realign the talus and the navicular bones in the ankle and foot, which are critical to the alignment and function of the ankle, knee, and hip. I told him to let his ankle relax and that he would feel a tug on his leg, which should not be painful. The adjustment brought the bones into a better biomechanical position. I repeated the shock-absorption test by pounding quite firmly on the bottom of his left foot. When I immediately retested the gluteus medius hip muscle, it now stayed on—it tested strong and felt much stronger to him.

Tom was truly impressed at the obvious improvement in function of his body following the correction of a twenty-five-year-old misalignment of his ankle. He wondered, "Why would anyone not do this? It's simple, it's safe, it's noninvasive, and it improves the function of the body. Even if someone still needed surgery or already had one, it is still critical to restore normal function—perhaps even more so if they already had a surgery. I am getting a picture of what you mean by healthcare, and maybe it is integrative medicine. Patients deserve the best from all worlds in healthcare."

Integrative healthcare doesn't mean abandoning what you already know and do for your body. It means expanding your perspective and recognizing that most chronic conditions are not diseases at all but modifiable conditions if you address the malfunctioning mechanisms that create them. But it requires thinking functionally when your body has a symptom, and analyzing body function. That's why Applied Kinesiology and diagnostic muscle testing are so significant. They allow providers to evaluate the function of your body in an immediate and practical way. They are changing the face of healthcare by providing a whole new form of doctor-patient interactive assessment.

Front-end alignment for a knee

Back to Tom. Having corrected his pelvis and ankle, I next wanted to look at the alignment of the knee itself. I tested the quadriceps (the front thigh muscle) because it supports the knee itself. The left quadriceps tested strong and obviously was on. I explained that I was then going to evaluate the knee alignment by testing the mechanoreceptor nerve endings in the knee ligaments. Since his tibia (lower leg) was rotated internally, which was stressing the joint surface on the medial side, I then challenged the knee ligaments by pushing his lower leg further into internal rotation and then retesting the quadriceps. When I did, it tested much weaker. The quadriceps is a very strong muscle, yet Tom could no longer hold his leg up against my testing pressure.

I wanted to do one more test to confirm what I suspected. This time I challenged the ligaments differently, rotating his lower leg in the opposite direction, turning it outwardly. I then retested the quadriceps. Following the outward rotation of the tibia, the quadriceps tested extremely strong. It was obviously on, once again. That confirmed the internal rotational misalignment of the lower leg, which I had seen without even a test. But the test told me that when his lower leg further internally rotates, the knee-supporting muscles shut off. And when his lower leg externally rotates, the muscles turn on. The problem is that his knee is misaligned such that the lower leg is internally rotated and probably has been that way since he sprained it twenty years ago. The pronation of his left foot and the misalignment of the pelvis further accentuated the internal rotation of the tibia.

With a normally functioning knee, I could challenge it in any direction and the knee-supporting muscles would stay on. A common misalignment like Tom's makes the knee vulnerable to reinjury. If he had tried running, each step on that pronated ankle would have increased the internal rotation and shut off the knee muscles. A turning motion, like changing directions, could have increased the misalignment and caused his knee to give out. He was fortunate that he never re-injured it in a major way.

With corrections to his knee's function, Tom can once again make exercise his ally. He will have to limit high-impact sports due to the existing loss of knee-joint surface, but he can be much more active with a reasonably healthy left knee. He won't have to worry anymore about his knee giving out on him if he moves the wrong way. The alignment and the muscles will support it.

I adjusted the left knee into proper alignment and then retested the quadriceps, which tested as being on. To re-challenge the knee, I firmly pushed the knee joint in every possible direction and retested the quadriceps each time. The quadriceps continued to stay on, no matter how hard or in what direction the knee was forced. I was satisfied that, now, if Tom's knee got twisted, it probably wouldn't shut off the supporting muscles.

Tom finally understood that my use of muscle testing wasn't about trying to strengthen weak muscles. I use it to evaluate and treat body function to improve the circuitry of the body so that muscles turn on and off properly during activity. Corrections normalize the function of the nervous system so it precisely and accurately controls the muscles, which then support the joints.

Our next and important task was to further normalize the function of the muscles that support his knee. If his body had them shut off for reasons other than the structural components we had just dealt with, we would have to work with his glandular system or other body functions to ensure normal support of the knee.

Looking at Tom through Chemical Spectacles

Tom, ever the medical doctor, looked taken aback: "Now you've lost me again. I was following this all very closely and thought I had it. What does my glandular system have to do with my knee?"

I made the point that science is learning much about the interconnectedness of the body and relationships between specific muscles and specific organs. Tom was familiar with viscerosomatic and somatovisceral reflexes—neurological terms that describe relationships wherein muscles share certain reflex pathways with specific organs. In viscerosomatic reflexes, a malfunction of an organ can reflexively cause a specific associated muscle to shut off. Whatever joint that shut off muscle should be supporting can become unstable or weak, producing symptoms such as weak or painful joints that appear to be structural or mechanical in nature.

Up to this point, Tom and I had dealt with muscles being shut off by faulty mechanoreceptors from ligaments or from the muscles themselves. For each, a physical trauma or injury had upset the normal function of the nerve endings. And for each, I was able to reset them through mechanical adjustments that realigned a joint, such as his pelvis, ankle, and knee. I reset his ankle muscles by manipulative corrections on the origins and insertions (where the muscles attach to the bones). In other words, I had thus far treated muscles that were shut off specifically due to structural problems. But I suspected that dysfunctioning organs were shutting off some of his knee muscles. We would have to deal with that for him to have the full support for his knee.

Tom wondered why I suspected he had dysfunctioning organs and reminded me that he was seeing me for his knee problem. I told him that my suspicion was based on a combination of the medical history he'd provided, his medial knee pain, and my observations of his foot pronation and specific pelvic misalignment. These types of problems are commonly caused by a lack of support from muscles that are each related to the adrenal glands. It certainly didn't mean he had disease of his adrenal glands, but his history indicated a strong possibility of adrenal dysfunction.

My plan was to individually test the major muscles that support the knee. If any were turned off, the next step would be to test to determine the malfunction in his body causing them to be shut off.

Proceeding with the manual muscle tests of his knee-supporting muscles, two muscles tested very weak. They were clearly shut off. Several other muscles probably would have tested weak had I tested them before correcting the misaligned bones in his ankle. The fact that the two muscles were still shut off, even after basic mechanical corrections that corrected the other muscles, confirmed my suspicion of a need to look further. The next task was to address those two muscles, the sartorius and the gracilis. Because they run from the pelvis to the inside of the knee, their normal function is critical for supporting the medial collateral ligament and for preventing the knee from rotating inward, the exact way in which Tom's was injured. It was possible those muscles were already off, before the knee strain, and may have contributed to the injury by allowing it to twist excessively, leading to it giving out.

Those two muscles, commonly associated with adrenal gland function, represent a pattern I had seen hundreds of times, because it affects so many people. And as is often the case, it was probably affecting much more than just Tom's knee. Combined with his history of fatigue, knee inflammation, poor protein digestion, and even depression, the likely common denominator was the function of his adrenal glands.

Let's look at some basic adrenal functions—and at the saber-toothed tiger. Many baby boomers are ex-adrenaline junkies, people who lived in the fast lane for too many years. As they age, they are starting to have many of the same problems. Remember what happens when a tiger attacks the body or when any form of immediate stress occurs. In the fight-or-flight response, the sympathetic nervous system fires, releasing adrenal gland hormones to create survival mechanisms: elevated blood pressure and blood sugar, increased heart rate, dilated pupils, and opened-up air passageways (bronchodilation). On the other hand, the parasympathetic nervous system, which regulates day-to-day activities like slowing the heart rate and stimulating digestion, is inhibited. Normal digestion and even intestinal peristalsis is stopped to allow the body to focus on survival. As mentioned in chapter 1, an estimated 90 percent of visits to all types of doctors are for stress-related illnesses, and these are all caused by some variation of this imbalance.

Why the high blood pressure?

Prolonged activation of the stress response creates many chronic symptoms that accelerate aging and result in degenerative diseases. As discussed earlier, producing high amounts of adrenaline, for example, creates imbalance in the body, depletes the body of nutrients, and diminishes the body's ability to produce more adrenaline in the future. Dr. Hans Selye, a pioneer in the field of stress research, referred to three stages the adrenal glands progress through when frequently and repeatedly activated by stress.[1] He termed these stages the General Adaptation Syndrome. The initial stress response, the

Alarm Stage, is the classic fight-or-flight response that brings on a rush of adrenaline.

Selye observed that when laboratory animals were stressed repeatedly and continuously, their bodies went into the Resistance Stage. If you are under prolonged stress, the resistance stage may last years or even decades, during which several changes take place in your body. One is an enlargement of the outer layer of the adrenal glands (the cortex), where hormones are produced that control mineral balance, blood-sugar levels, inflammation, and even secondary sex characteristics. During the resistance stage, Selye's animals developed stomach and intestinal ulcers as well as a shrinking of the thymus gland and lymphatic system, leading to a weakening of their immune systems. In humans, this explains the enormous increase of digestive problems such as heartburn, GERD, irritable bowel syndrome, as well as the chronic illnesses and fatigue so often found in people subjected to ongoing stress.

At some point, the body can no longer maintain the increased production of these hormones to meet the continued, ongoing stress, and the adrenals reach the Exhaustion Stage, wherein the body can no longer regulate its own vital functions.

Because the stress mechanisms and the adrenal glands control so many functions in the body, they are a factor in a wide variety of chronic health problems.

Tom and I contrasted our different approaches. His approach to help a patient with high blood pressure would be to prescribe at least one or two blood-pressure medications, including a diuretic, to bring the blood pressure down. But in my search for a cause for the elevated blood pressure, I would look at the mechanisms by which the body controls its own blood pressure, such as its control of mineral balance and dilation versus constriction of the blood vessels. For instance, aldosterone is produced by the adrenal cortex and causes the body to retain sodium and water. If your adrenal glands are being stimulated to produce excess aldosterone, your blood pressure would likely be elevated. In the TWM treatment of people who have high blood pressure, it is a fairly common practice to give a medication that blocks the effect of aldosterone, so it won't make the body retain excess salt and water. It isn't used on everyone with elevated blood pressure, and it doesn't lower everyone's blood pressure, because not everyone with hypertension has it due to an excess of aldosterone. But if they do, giving them medication to block aldosterone will typically lower their blood pressure. That is one approach.

The holistic approach is to question why a person's aldosterone level is too high to begin with. As discussed earlier, you can have too much of a chemical in your body either because you produce too much or don't break it down efficiently. Since the liver normally breaks down aldosterone, an excess of aldosterone may be due to a sluggish liver. The sluggishness and inability of the liver to efficiently break down aldosterone can be due to excessive amounts of refined sugar, alcohol, caffeine, or bad fats in the diet; to lack of exercise; or even to a deficiency of B vitamins, which the liver uses to break down aldosterone. So improving liver function, or addressing a malfunctioning liver, may help allow the body to regulate its own blood pressure.

The question is what is the best way to deal with the imbalance of the Inner Pharmacy so the body can regulate itself with its own mechanisms, without medication. If the imbalance is too severe or advanced, it may require the external pharmacy to control the blood pressure, but why ignore the body's own mechanisms and ability to regulate itself?

To normalize the Inner Pharmacy, a holistic approach, as always, looks not just at the symptom but at the person with the elevated blood pressure. As a doctor-and-patient team, you look at the person's relationship to stress, what he eats and drinks, how he exercises, and what he does or doesn't do to offset effects of stress. If you can improve the function of the body and influence these factors, there is a reasonable chance of improving his blood pressure.

Chiropractic and osteopathic adjustments can effectively influence the function of the liver, the adrenals, and the kidneys, all of which contribute to the control of blood pressure in the body. Stimulating the parasympathetic nerves through cranial and sacral corrections can favor the dilation of blood vessels, versus the constriction that occurs from the sympathetic nervous system's stress response. Nutrients such as calcium, magnesium, vitamin E, riboflavin, and essential fatty acids can help reduce blood pressure. These can all help shift the body's Inner Pharmacy so it can control its own blood pressure.

Unfortunately, many people's mechanisms to control their blood pressure are so deteriorated or imbalanced that lifestyle changes and conservative treatment have only limited effect. Fortunately, medications exist which will control blood pressure. But the value is clear in addressing the body's own blood-pressure controlling mechanisms. At the very least, improving body function may help you be more healthy in general and perhaps require less medication or delay the need for additional medications.

Tom and I agreed, wholeheartedly, that the best approach to controlling blood pressure would be an integrated approach that normalizes the function of the Inner Pharmacy first and then uses external pharmaceuticals second as a way of augmenting the Inner Pharmacy.

Recognizing adrenal dysfunction

Getting back to the doctor and his knee, remember that I was alerted to his adrenal glands by his symptoms and the involvement of two specific medial knee-supporting muscles. I proceeded to ask him a couple of questions. I asked if bright light bothered his eyes.

He replied that he squints and sometimes gets a headache unless he wears sunglasses outside. He also wondered what that meant to me.

I had observed that his pupils are quite large and dilated, which is a common body-language pattern of adrenal dysfunction. I also asked if he ever felt dizzy from standing up fast.

His response was that sometimes he did. Like most people, and not thinking functionally, he just assumed that it was normal and that he stood up too fast. However, since this is another sign of adrenal dysfunction, I wanted to check his blood pressure. He was a bit reluctant, and he said he could almost guarantee that it would not be high. He informed me that, on the contrary, "it's usually lower than normal."

I told him that this is what I suspected and that I wasn't so concerned about what his blood pressure was. I wanted to see what it did when he changed positions. First, I checked it with him lying down on his back. Then, I had him stand up, and I immediately checked it again. The systolic, the top number of a blood-pressure reading, should rise from six to ten millimeters of pressure. That normal rise results from a good level of adrenal chemicals causing a constriction of the abdominal blood vessels so the blood gets up to the head. It takes more pressure to get the blood up to your head when you are standing than when you are lying down. If you don't get that immediate rise in blood pressure with standing, which is usually the case when people feel dizzy upon standing, it probably means that your adrenals are underactive or depleted.

His top number didn't rise with standing. In fact, it dropped six. Since that is what is happening when he gets up from lying and perhaps, to a lesser degree, from sitting, it explains his frequent dizziness upon standing. It also gave me a baseline that measured one aspect of adrenal dysfunction. I knew that if I could improve the health of his adrenal glands so his Inner Pharmacy could produce more normal amounts of certain adrenal chemicals, there would be a normal rise with standing in the future.

He found this simple functional test and its significance to be quite interesting. I was testing his blood pressure, not just to see what it *is*, but *what it does*. It reflects the status of the adrenal glands, and it is a rather obvious test to do if you want to measure function. I explained that I might want to do some additional laboratory tests of blood and saliva to assess the levels of various hormones, but for the moment we could proceed with the data we had. With his low blood pressure that dropped even further when he stood up, it was unlikely that he currently had underactive adrenals. From his history, symptoms, and my observations, I was fairly sure his body was somewhere late in the resistance stage of the general adaptation syndrome.

To understand what that means, realize that *the early part of the resistance stage* may go on for years, depending on how long someone is able to maintain a level of overactivity of their stress mechanisms. And that is determined by factors such as the frequency and intensity of the stress, the inherent genetic strength of a person's adrenal glands, their nutritional status, and their personal attitudes about stress and lifestyle factors about stress reduction. It is not unusual for people to develop health problems during this stage due to the glandular and nervous-system imbalance. Depending on their biochemical individuality and how well they handle stress, they may develop high blood pressure, digestive or inflammatory problems, or blood-sugar handling problems. Even if they don't develop obvious symptoms that catch their attention at this stage, the imbalance in "inflammation-regulating chemicals" is probably allowing for the slow, insidious development of coronary heart disease or maybe degenerative arthritis, depending on their genetic predispositions.

Nevertheless, a point is reached where the body can no longer maintain the excess production of stress chemicals, and the previously overactive adrenal glands then become underactive. They are fatigued and often depleted of nutrient building blocks they need to produce the emergency stress hormones. Because the adrenals produce so many different chemicals and regulate so many activities, these various functions can fatigue at different rates, producing different problems depending on the individual. It is all part of each person's biochemical uniqueness.

High-adrenaline lifestyles just can't last forever. Some people experience an abrupt breakdown of one of their "stress-regulating" mechanisms, and they "crash and burn" with an intense health crisis. Other people, more like the doctor, experience a gradual breakdown and may have a variety of migrating symptoms. But most significantly, they just don't feel great and no longer feel like themselves. There is often a stressful event preceding this shift. It's like an exaggerated adrenal "letdown." Remember a stressful time when you had to push yourself hard to meet a certain deadline. Many people can relate to a time in school when they had term papers due and final exams. They pushed themselves hard, used a lot of extra adrenaline, and did what it took to meet the deadlines. After exams and once the saber-toothed tiger was no longer chasing them, they probably collapsed out of exhaustion. That's the "letdown" of the adrenals once the immediate threat is over. That is also when many people get sick, or their back "goes out" on them, or some other problem develops.

Usually a few days of rest and relaxation rejuvenates the adrenals. Yet people eventually reach a point where they no longer bounce back like they used to, or they develop a problem that the body can no longer simply self-correct. That is usually when their adrenals are run-down and underactive.

I took a wild guess that the doctor had had a high-adrenaline lifestyle for years preceding his knee injury. If he was anything like most doctors, he was likely a "type A" high-achieving individual who had pushed himself hard during high school, college, and graduate school. During medical school, he probably didn't have the healthiest diet or any major stress-reduction program, and somewhere along the line he stopped all exercise except basketball, which is primarily anaerobic. At that point, he was the classic weekend warrior: highly stressed with a low level of fitness but loving the adrenaline rush and fun of playing basketball. What he didn't realize was that his lifestyle kept him constantly running from a saber-toothed tiger, and when he played basketball, his run intensified to a sprint. Like many people, he was somewhat of an adrenaline "junkie."

Tom agreed that this bit of conjecture described him well. He said it was a bit scary to hear his life described this way, and he realized that he really was an accident looking for a place to happen.

Chances are that his body shut off those adrenal-related knee muscles due to his adrenal fatigue. I suspect they were already shut off and allowed his knee to twist, thus contributing to his knee injury. Since he had experienced the bad ankle sprain five years earlier, the ankle was probably shutting off some other important knee muscles upon impact of the foot. It's most likely that he actually had several malfunctions weakening his knee at that time. And that is so often why joints give out on people. More significant, his knee never healed on its own. In twenty years, it never regained its normal alignment and function, and it continued to deteriorate.

Rebuilding the adrenal glands

If we could get Tom's whole body functioning better and rebuild his adrenals, there was a good chance those adrenal-related knee muscles would turn on properly and stay on. Rebuilding his adrenals would likely also improve his digestion and lessen his fatigue, depression, and inflammation.

He was excited about the potential benefits but questioned if it was possible to actually "rebuild the adrenal glands." It isn't a quick fix, but yes, it can usually be done. Long-term health benefits accumulate as the glands repair and rebuild themselves and return to more normal function. The healing power of nature works, given the opportunity. His adrenals had probably been trying to repair themselves for over twenty years but hadn't been able to, perhaps because he continued to be attacked by saber-toothed tigers and his adrenals never got the chance to rest. While that may have been part of it, I suspected there was more going on. Overstimulating the adrenals not only exhausts them, it also depletes many nutrients they use as raw materials to make various adrenal hormones.

Two important ingredients used to make adrenaline are vitamin B-6 and the amino acid tyrosine. If your body needs to produce one thousand times the normal amount of adrenaline, you will need one thousand times the amount of B-6 and tyrosine to do it, and a deficiency of raw materials is one of the ways that high-adrenaline lifestyles get people into trouble. Their bodies simply run out of raw materials. Though the body can manufacture its own tyrosine from other amino acids, something becomes compromised and eventually depleted from the exponential increase in its utilization. Remember, for our ancestors, a saber-toothed tiger attack was an occasional event. It didn't happen every day, much less many times a day.

I highly suspected that Tom was deficient in several of the B vitamins and perhaps in tyrosine. Before testing for these, I explained that for his adrenals to successfully heal, the building-up process would have to take place faster than the tearing-down process. Several changes in his lifestyle were needed, nothing difficult, but they would require attention and discipline on his part. I could do certain critical parts of the process, but I couldn't do it all. I had to know that he was willing to make diet and lifestyle changes that would support the rebuilding of his adrenal glands. Needless to say, lifestyle change was much more than Tom anticipated when he consulted with me for his knee problem, but he was ready to make the changes. He could see the need for them.

Parts of my treatment to improve his knee could be likened to resetting adrenal "circuit breakers," which had been off since being overloaded years ago. I could reset them, but I couldn't stop Tom from overloading them again. Only he could do that. If he didn't do his part, I'd be resetting them forever and Tom would make little progress in improving his overall health.

The point is, patients are not dependent on their doctor to make them well. On the contrary, I guide people like Tom in ways to sustain their health with a minimum of future input from me.

With a mutual understanding of the doctor-patient relationship, it was time to consider specific possibilities to improve the nutrient status of Tom's adrenal glands. Nutrients are different from drugs. A drug is a substance given for its effect on a specific organ or type of cell in the body. Mainstream doctors often use drugs as "replacement" therapy: if the body is unable to produce enough of a specific chemical, a pharmaceutical form of that chemical is prescribed. This replaces what the body isn't able to produce on its own.

At times, replacement therapy is appropriate and necessary. It is, however, grossly overused. It is frequently not the only option and by itself usually does not strengthen the gland that should be producing the chemical. More often than not, it has a weakening effect, the gland atrophies, and the drug has created a dependence in which the person now needs it to function.

A nutrient, however, is a food substance that supplies the molecular building blocks or cofactors the body needs to produce chemicals on its own. For example, the adrenal glands make adrenaline from an amino acid, a protein called tyrosine, and it is known that one factor affecting adrenaline production is the blood level of tyrosine. I suspected that Tom, like many people, had a stress-induced depletion of adrenaline and its close cousin, noradrenaline. The Inner Pharmacy can limit production of these and other vital neurotransmitters if it doesn't have enough raw materials and also if the adrenals are fatigued from years of excess adrenaline production.

Here's an example of the role of the adrenal glands in asthma. If either Tom or I were treating a patient with asthma, we would each want to improve bronchodilation (the opening up of air passageways in the lungs). He would do that by prescribing pharmaceutical forms of adrenaline and perhaps other adrenal hormones that dilate the bronchioles and open the air passageways to improve breathing.

My strategy would be similar: relieve the asthma by improving bronchodilation through increased adrenal chemicals. The difference is that I would do this by helping the body produce more of the bronchodilating chemicals on its own by improving the function of the patient's adrenal glands and by providing more of the nutrients needed by the patient's body to increase its production of the needed chemicals. If the patient's Inner Pharmacy can produce more bronchodilators, then the asthma gets better, purely based on improved body function. As the body heals and gets stronger in its own ability to produce bronchodilating chemicals, the patient becomes less dependent on the inhalers and other medications. Again, there is great value in normalizing the Inner Pharmacy as the first choice.

Of course, I am not suggesting you stop taking a medication you need. I am, however, paying great attention and respect for the body's ability to heal and regulate itself, when given the opportunity. The body's Inner Pharmacy is light-years ahead of our most advanced understanding of biochemistry and pharmacology. My goal is to restore normal physiology so the healing power of nature can do its work.

Tom agreed that, in the asthma example, if we combined our approaches, we could get the best results for many asthma patients. Western medicine could provide the chemicals an asthma sufferer's body needs, while a holistic approach works to improve function so the person can eventually produce those chemicals themselves.

This team approach works for people with high blood pressure, heart disease, arthritis, mood disorders, and other chronic conditions, even the early stages of diabetes. The economic impact, alone, of lessening reliance on pharmaceuticals would provide great relief for individuals, insurance companies, and government-funded programs that pay for medications.

Back to the doctor's knee problem. I repeated the manual muscle tests of the two muscles that had tested weak. Since they still tested weak, we agreed that whatever we had done up to this point had not changed them and that, as they were, they would not provide much support to the damaged medial side of his knee.

Then I placed a small amount of tyrosine on Tom's tongue and gave him a few seconds to taste it. I wanted to see if stimulating the nerve endings on his tongue with a nutrient I thought his adrenal glands needed would turn on the adrenal-related muscle.

I then retested the muscle. There was an immediate strengthening. This previously weak knee-supporting muscle was now clearly facilitated. To Tom, it felt like I wasn't even applying pressure during the second test. But he realized I was using significant force, and the muscle felt totally different. He didn't have to strain or shift his body to keep his leg in position; it was almost effortless, as it should be when a muscle is on and doing its job.

"Could the tyrosine on my tongue make such a huge difference?" he asked.

"It's like flipping a switch," I explained. The switch was in his nervous system, and the presence of the tyrosine addressed a deficiency in his body that was causing the muscle to be switched off. Chances are that the muscle inhibition was due to an autonomic nervous system reflex resulting from a lack of available tyrosine which was limiting his body's production of adrenal-related chemicals. The muscle tested and felt stronger because it was being properly turned on by his nervous system when it got the signal (from his tongue) that tyrosine was on the way.

If we were to rinse his mouth to remove the tyrosine from his tongue, the muscle weakness would return. It would shut off again.

"So what am I supposed to do?" joked the doctor. "Keep tyrosine on my tongue forever?"

"No," I replied. As Tom increased his dietary intake of tyrosine, his body could replenish its storage and use it to make the chemicals it needs so that the adrenal-related muscle will begin to stay on.

Since his Inner Pharmacy needed to make the necessary hormones and neurotransmitters, I suggested that Tom also supplement his diet with additional new materials for the adrenals, such as niacin, folic acid, B-6, and vitamin C.

You are "what your body does with" what you eat

I wanted to do more treatment to help normalize Tom's adrenal function and bring more balance to his autonomic nervous system. It's not simply a matter of providing the body with necessary nutrients; it's also a matter of getting the body to do the right things with the raw materials. The treatment helps to reset the circuit breakers. The nutrients then help the adrenal glands to function better so the circuit breakers stay reset. If he just took the nutrients and did nothing else, the circuit breakers might eventually reset themselves. But I could do it with precision and predictability by using the data I had and the muscles as indicators. If the muscles stayed on, I knew the circuit was working—which meant that Tom's knee would be more stable and probably that his adrenal function was improving. If the muscles tested weak or "shut off" again, I would know that something was still missing or perhaps that he was still tearing his adrenals down faster than we were building them up. We would also know that his knee was still vulnerable to injury and could give out from the lack of muscle support.

How could Tom have gotten so deficient in tyrosine? The first reason was Tom's high-adrenaline lifestyle in his twenties. The second was that he might not have been getting enough tyrosine or its ingredients from his diet. Tyrosine is an amino acid, a protein that can come directly from foods. The body can also produce it from another amino acid called phenylalanine, which the body must obtain from proteins in the diet. Tom had said he didn't digest proteins well and had avoided high-protein foods for a long time. Chances are he simply wasn't supplying his body with enough tyrosine and other amino acids, either because he was not consuming enough protein or he wasn't properly digesting the proteins he did consume. Compounded by the excess production of adrenal hormones, he was using up more than he was able to replenish.

Tyrosine is sometimes referred to as the "antidepressant" amino acid. People deficient in tyrosine tend to become depressed as well as fatigued. Besides the adrenal hormones, tyrosine is also used in the body's production of thyroid hormone. A lack of available tyrosine is not a good thing, since it is needed to produce hormones that normally help you feel "up," and a deficiency predisposes you to feel depressed and to develop mood disorders.

When Tom mentioned the depression that began after his knee injury, I suspected that he developed a tyrosine deficiency around that time, probably when his adrenals entered the downside of the resistance stage. If he was low in tyrosine, it not only contributed to his knee weakness and lack of healing, it probably also contributed to years of depression. The fact that he experienced improvement from antidepressant medication supports the hypothesis that his depression was due to a chemical imbalance, an imbalance that can be corrected by helping Tom's Inner Pharmacy produce more of its own antidepressants.

In the discussion of Selye's General Adaptation Syndrome in chapter 5, I noted that is common to develop digestive problems during the resistance stage. The continued activation of the sympathetic nervous system by ongoing bouts of stress puts the body into survival mode. Normal digestive processes are inhibited while the body tries to survive the current crisis. As the crisis goes on and on, the body's normal production of digestive enzymes continues to be "shut off" or greatly reduced. So when people eat heavier foods, such as proteins that require more enzymes to break them down, and the enzymes aren't there, it creates discomfort: bloating, gas, and heartburn. This is exactly what Tom described when he told me why he avoids protein foods.

Unfortunately, rather than looking for the cause of these common digestive disorders, we have been programmed to take an antacid or medication for "immediate relief" of our symptoms. While we may experience temporary relief, this approach rarely corrects the imbalance in the nervous system that is limiting our normal digestion. Many people constantly take medications for stomach discomfort and think that the problem is gone because they no longer feel it.

A better approach is to treat the imbalance in the nervous system to allow the parasympathetics to stimulate normal digestive activity.

It can be reset through chiropractic or osteopathic corrections and perhaps lifestyle changes to make for a permanent improvement.

In Tom's history, he told me he takes medication to decrease stomach-acid production and that it also helped to reduce his heart-burn. Hearing this, I knew it would be good to look at his diaphragm function to make sure it was doing its job in keeping the acid in the stomach and out of his esophagus. His hunched shoulders and tight abdominals also alerted me to the strong possibility of a diaphragm problem, and correcting his diaphragm muscle could be critical to restoring normal digestive function.

But first I wanted to make sure Tom understood the importance of normal protein intake and digestion. Poor digestion likely contributed to his depression by limiting his tyrosine availability, and low proteins probably accelerated the deterioration of the joint surface of his knee.

Preserving your joints with protein

The association of knee pain, joint surfaces, digestion, and protein intake caught Tom off guard, but again it forced him to think more functionally. He would have looked closely at skeletons and cadavers in medical school, so I began to discuss the appearance and feel of articulating cartilage (the surface of a joint where one bone meets another). In many older skeletons and cadavers, those joint surfaces, which are supposed to be very smooth, are quite rough in texture. It is amazing that weight-bearing joints, such as knees, ankles, hips, and spinal joints, work as well as they do for as long as they do. The smoothness of the joint surface is a critical factor that allows one bone to glide over another. In young people and those with healthy joints, the surface of a joint is one of the smoothest things found in nature. That smooth surface also contains a high concentration of protein, many times over the protein concentration of the circulating blood. If your body is deficient in protein, joint surfaces deteriorate more rapidly. Besides lacking the protein to sustain the smoothness of the joint, protein can also be robbed from the protein-rich joint sur-faces to be used elsewhere in the body.

When a joint surface loses protein, it loses its smoothness. Over time, the joint surface can change from the smoothness of polished marble to the roughness of sandpaper. That is the degenerative process which underlies osteoarthritis, the wear and tear type of arthritis, and it is greatly accelerated by a protein deficiency.

Good protein levels and good joint biomechanics, including proper alignment, muscle support during activity, and proper shock absorption, can slow degeneration. Glucosamine and purified chondroitin sulfates (available as supplements) can be helpful in slowing the degeneration of joint surfaces because they provide ingredients for the repair and rebuilding of cartilage. Good dietary protein and normal protein digestion contribute to this process in a very fundamental way.

Do I recommend high-protein diets for everyone? Following the general rule that "there is a time and place for everything," high-protein diets, as do other specialty diets, have their place. They can help many people lose weight and can provide an abundance of ingredients for building muscle. But they are not usually "health-promoting" when used for extended times. For one thing, high-protein diets create extra work for the kidneys. For another thing, it is very difficult to maintain healthy ratios of the pro- and anti-inflammatory chemicals called prostaglandins that are made from dietary fats. I talked about these ratios when I described Ellen and her inflammation in chapter 4. Unless most of your high-protein diet is from fish, there is going to be an abundance of a chemical called arachadonic acid, which encourages inflammation in the body. In some people, you may not see it until they have been on a high-protein diet for a few years. But the shift toward greater inflammation usually comes at some point.

For most people, I recommend a moderate-protein diet with a balance of good-quality proteins. Consuming proteins with high-carbohydrate foods also interferes with protein digestion for most people, so a good rule of thumb is to have protein along with vegetables but not with starches, fruits, or sweets. This contradicts standard ideas about meat and potatoes, but meat is much better digested if consumed with a salad and vegetables. Simply reducing starches, pastas, and other high-carbohydrate foods also goes a long way toward helping people take off extra pounds.

In Tom's situation, I was fairly confident he needed more protein and less carbohydrate in his diet. He didn't need to lose weight. I arranged for a blood test the next day to obtain a baseline of his protein levels. As for deficiency in tyrosine, I couldn't tell him to add more protein to his diet to remedy it, since his body wasn't able to digest protein well. Addressing his deficiency would require corrections first to improve his digestive function and then addressing his diet.

He was relieved that I wasn't going to change his diet without doing something to improve his ability to digest it. He understood the protein relationship to his knee and the need for normal digestion. He was willing to take the tyrosine supplement and to eat more protein from different sources to get a variety of amino acids, as long as his digestive system cooperated. He was hopeful it would improve his energy level and his depression as well as slow the degeneration of his knee.

It's not about the weight

He did question why he, a skinny person, needed to limit carbohydrates. I explained that it had little to do with weight and build. One concern is that a high-carbohydrate diet acts to sustain carbohydrate metabolism. Since Tom primarily consumed carbohydrate foods, that is what his body burned for fuel. Recall that with Ellen, we improved her running endurance by improving her fat metabolism. I encouraged her to shift from carbohydrate metabolism, which produces short bursts of energy, to fat metabolism, which produces a more sustained energy that supports endurance. As Ellen decreased her carbohydrate intake, consumed more protein and good fat, took capsules of fish oil, and monitored her heart rate to optimize her fat metabolism, her endurance improved and her inflammation disappeared.

Watching Tom, I could see how fatigued he was getting, as he hadn't eaten for a few hours. It appeared that his carbohydrate diet was fueling him for only a few hours, and then low blood sugar made him feel fatigued and foggy. He may have even been getting a reactive hypoglycemia, in which the body reacts to carbohydrate intake by producing too much insulin, which then excessively lowers the level of sugar in the blood. This is another problem that wears down the adrenal glands. When the blood-sugar level is dropping or going low, the adrenals' normal response is to counter that drop and elevate the blood sugar by releasing a glucocorticoid hormone called cortisol.

The problem is that cortisol is a stress hormone. Cortisol not only increases blood sugar, it also increases blood pressure and blood clotting. It creates anxiety, suppresses the immune system, prevents many people from falling asleep, and wakens them during the night. In producing high amounts of cortisol, the body also uses up many of the same raw materials it could otherwise use to produce non-stress, vital hormones like DHEA and testosterone. Naturally, an ongoing high cortisol production further depletes the adrenal glands and works against the rebuilding process that is so essential.

Along with his diet changes, Tom needed to start some aerobic exercise on a regular basis to help him shift to more fat metabolism, which would help his energy, mood, excess inflammation, and endurance. He agreed to get a heart-rate monitor and to follow the aerobic formula explained in chapter 4.

A fat myth

Tom did have one other concern, a common one for people embarking on such a diet change. He was worried that eating more fat might make him fat and that it might raise his cholesterol. Both are common misconceptions. I explained that when he eats a plate of pasta, approximately 40 percent of it gets converted to fat and stored in the body. Just because he had been on a low-fat diet did not mean that his body had no fat. In his history, Tom mentioned that blood tests showed him to have elevated triglycerides, which usually stems from an excess consumption of alcohol or carbohydrate. So, unless he had a high alcohol consumption that he hadn't told me about, the high triglycerides meant he was eating more carbohydrates than he was burning up. His body was converting the excess carbohydrate into fat and transporting it in the blood to storage sites.

Having elevated triglycerides means that your blood is much thicker than it should be, that is, it is more the consistency of cream rather than water, as it should be. I once had a patient who had very elevated triglycerides. After spinning the blood down to separate it, the serum, which normally looks like apple juice, had the consistency of lard. It was almost solid. I doubted that Tom's triglycerides were that high. But any elevation makes the blood thicker, requires the heart to pump harder, and means there are more fats in the cardiovascular system. And that is all from a low-fat diet!

Eating a balanced diet with more good fat will not make you fat, especially if you train your body to burn fat through aerobic exercise. It will probably even improve the ratio of good and bad cholesterols so that your cardiovascular risk ratio improves over what it was on the low-fat diet. It is usually easy to normalize elevated triglycerides and can often be done in a matter of weeks. It may require doing something to improve liver function, but Tom's triglycerides would probably come down nicely if he reduced his carbohydrate intake and started exercising to burn more calories and fat.

As for low-carbohydrates, a diet fad then in vogue, most people missed the mark, as usual, by dwelling on the minutiae of the diet and how many low-carb desserts they could get away with. It would be so much better if we would just focus on eating a balance of healthy, nutrient-rich foods.

But the core idea of low-carbohydrate diets has merit. I often recommend it to patients because, in moderation, it makes sense and is a low-stress diet for the body. It is a good diet for "ex-adrenaline junkies" to rebuild their adrenals, which can then help with headaches, back pain, knee pain, fatigue, digestive problems, inflammation, and so on. I recommend that diet because mechanical corrections often respond better if people aren't subjecting themselves to huge deviations in their blood-sugar levels during the course of a day. When done properly and in moderation, a low-carbohydrate diet works.

Remember, diet is a tool to sustain your lifestyle and improve your health. No one diet is right for everyone at all times. Someone doing hard physical work for eight hours a day has a different set of requirements than someone sitting at a desk those same eight hours. And someone under constant attack from a saber-toothed tiger has different dietary requirements than someone sitting in a cave and meditating eight hours a day.

I put many of my patients on a diet, and it has nothing to do with losing weight. It just means eating healthful foods. It has to do with building the weak links in the body, helping repair injured areas, and—overall—improving their health and quality of life. Like Tom, many of us need some improvement in our body function so we can digest healthful food. Many of us also need some treatment to improve our body mechanics so we can be active, exercise properly, and receive the benefits of exercise. When I finish treating Tom and guiding him toward a healthy lifestyle, he will feel better than he has for many years. Yes, all of this will help to improve his knee. But even more important, it will help the person with the knee problem.

As a doctor, Tom was familiar with the "fight-or-flight" response of the autonomic nervous system. But like most of us, he had no idea how significantly it affects us in our everyday life. He didn't realize that years of high-stress living was creating such a distortion in his whole neuroendocrine system that it was even affecting his digestion.

When under constant attack by saber-toothed tigers, of course Tom's body would have to go into major adaptations for his own survival. It's not an exaggeration to say that under constant stress, anyone would eventually become weak in the knees. It is just a matter of applying knowledge of anatomy, physiology, and biomechanics to a functioning human being.

NSAIDs and your body's own anti-inflammatory chemicals

We needed to address one other aspect of chemical imbalance that had been adversely affecting Tom's digestive system: his almost daily use of non-steroidal anti-inflammatory drugs (NSAIDs) over the past twenty years. Examples of over-the-counter NSAIDs are aspirin, ibuprofen, naproxen, and ketoprofen. Prescription NSAIDs include higher-strength versions of these anti-inflammatory drugs plus COX-2 inhibitors. Not only can NSAIDs create gut problems and even interfere with normal fat metabolism, but stomach bleeding from their use is a leading cause of death in the United States, causing more deaths than AIDS.[2] And most of the time, there are no warning signs before serious problems develop. He knew this, but he tried not to think about it, and he knew of no other way to help his knee pain.

To shed light on American attitudes toward drugs and nutrients, I asked Tom if he had ever recommended that a patient take vitamin A. No, he said, he had not. He didn't know what to use it for and didn't know how much to use anyway. He also expressed concern that too much of it could be harmful.

It was a good and safe answer. But the fact is that deficiencies of vitamin A are quite common and can predispose you to problems with your skin and lymphatic system, as well as sinus and upper-respiratory infections and night-vision problems, to name a few. Yet people are afraid to take vitamin A. Sometimes it is because they don't know how much to take or what form to take it in. But there is a real fear that they might take too much and suffer irreparable damage.

I then asked Tom if he knew what happens when someone takes too much vitamin A. His vague response was, "Don't they get a headache?"

He was correct. They get a headache. As Linus Pauling, the Nobel Prize–winning biochemist once pointed out, no one has ever died from an overdose of vitamin A. Meanwhile, thousands of people die every year from aspirin and NSAIDs, and most people don't think twice about their risks and side effects. Sure, there is a harmful dose of vitamin A, and taking megadoses, such as over 50,000 IUs a day over long periods, can even cause liver damage. But no one is likely to do that. Vitamin A is not bad or risky to take. It is normally taken in the range of 2,500-5,000 IUs a day, and it helps the body create its own health.

Aspirin and NSAIDs are extremely useful in certain situations. But people grossly overuse them and underestimate their potential side effects.[3] Meanwhile, out of lack of knowledge, we are afraid to take vitamins and nutrients that could improve our health. However, even if you didn't take the perfect combination of vitamins, the side effects are relatively harmless and are a fraction of the harm done from misuse of over-the-counter medications.

Tom's use of NSAIDs was quite risky and may have damaged his digestive system over the past twenty years. It was going to take some work to get his Inner Pharmacy producing more of its own anti-inflammatory chemicals, but I thought it could be done with his cooperation in scheduling appointments and following through on the corrections. It would require him to change his diet, take recommended supplements, and add regular aerobic exercise and stress reduction.

I also recommended that he decrease and eventually eliminate his regular use of NSAIDs. As the corrections and lifestyle changes reduce the stress on his knee, he probably wouldn't need the medication much longer anyway. His knee pain reduced dramatically when I adjusted his pelvis, ankle, and knee and reset some of the supporting muscles. As his adrenal glands improved through rebuilding and repairing, other knee-supporting muscles would provide additional structural support and his adrenals would make more of their own anti-inflammatory chemicals.

The treatment

Next, I wanted to evaluate and, if necessary, treat his diaphragm to improve its function. Correcting it would help him to have more energy, breathe more deeply, and get more oxygen to his brain, and it may also help keep digestive acid and enzymes out of his esophagus. This would be an important piece to restoring normal digestive function. Then I planned to do some chiropractic corrections on his cranium and spine to stimulate the parasympathetic nerves to his stomach and digestive system so he could start digesting protein properly. He could take digestive enzymes to help his body break down protein, but we decided to wait on that option, since I would much rather correct the body so that it produces its own enzymes. The spinal corrections would also stimulate the nerve supply to the adrenal glands to assist in their healing.

The strategy was that when he leaves my office, the switches will be reset and the circuits will be on for normal function of his body. He will be able to eat protein without heartburn or stomach discomfort, and his knee-supporting muscles will all be "on" and working properly. I recommended that he see me again in a few days to test if all of this "holds," and chances are that some will have to be corrected or reset a few times. But the better job he does with his diet, exercise, supplements, and stress reduction, the faster this will

145

progress. I would get him molded for the orthotics to counter the foot pronation, and I would arrange for the blood tests we talked about. I also wanted to tape his left ankle to help hold up the arch and prevent the foot from pronating and the knee from turning in until his orthotics are made and can provide that support.

After hearing my recommendations, his comment was, "Let's do it." Tom felt like we were working together on this, and he was willing to do his part. In holistic healthcare, especially with regard to chronic conditions, you as a patient have a much greater role in the process, both in the choices and the responsibility to participate. This was all a new experience for Tom, and it was already changing his perspective of the doctor-patient relationship.

I proceeded to do the corrections and adjustments. I explained each step as I was doing corrections to improve his diaphragm and stomach, craniosacral mechanism, spine, and autonomic nervous system including adrenal gland function.

After doing the adjustments and corrections and before he got up from the examining table, I wanted to recheck his blood pressure first with him lying down and then immediately upon standing.

Remember that his top number *dropped* six when we measured it before treating him. This time it *came up* eight, which is a significant improvement and right in the normal range. That was an excellent response from his body, and it meant that his adrenal glands were already functioning better. Seeing that positive change in the positional blood pressure also helped me to know that the treatment was effective.

I then asked Tom to stand still, in front of me, so that I could reexamine his posture from behind and the side, comparing it with pre-treatment observations.

His alignment and posture were much improved. Not only were his legs now even in length when lying down, but his pelvis was also level when standing. He was less "knock-kneed," and his left foot was much less pronated. Even without the orthotics or taping, which I was about to do, his ankle muscles were supporting him much better. This was probably the first time in twenty-five years that those muscles were being properly turned on by his nervous system. He was also not as hunched over forward. He was breathing much more deeply, which meant better diaphragm function, better stomach function, more energy, and more oxygen to his brain.

Even though I routinely see such dramatic improvements from treating people, each time it is a delight. I reiterated that it was Tom's job to make the lifestyle changes that will help to maintain these corrections and to build on this new level of improved function. When I asked how he felt, he lightened up—literally and figuratively.

He felt light and centered, almost weightless, and was quite astounded that nothing hurt. This is how a body looks and feels when it is functioning properly.

"It's incredible. It's like the high I used to get, playing basketball. There's this clarity, like a fog has been lifted." He hesitated. "I'm afraid to move. Will I lose this feeling?"

I told him that he could move and that what I really wanted to accomplish was for his body to work well enough to not lose that feeling and even to be able to re-create some of it through normal activity.

"It's like the Fountain of Youth!" he laughed.

I didn't mean to burst his bubble, but some of the heightened awareness he was experiencing was a result of the stimulation his nervous system had just received from the adjustments and manipulations. The massive stimulation of nerve receptors sends a lot of information to your nervous system in a process called afferentation. His nervous system had not received normal stimulation from those receptors for a long time and was actually deficient in its function, a process referred to as dys-afferentation or sometimes as de-afferentation. The human nervous system loves stimulation, and much of it normally comes from the activation of nerve endings in joints when they move properly. Now with his joints better aligned and moving properly, Tom will reinforce this process as he gets more physically active and has more motion in his daily life.

The joy of a functioning body—and a good doctor/patient relationship

Tom wondered how I did it and if everyone felt this good after a treatment. I pointed out that it certainly takes a lot of study, training, practice, and a professional license. And yes, when the nervous system is stimulated properly, people usually experience an increased clarity and heightened awareness.

Like many of my patients, Tom noted that this had been different from any kind of doctor appointment he had ever experienced. Whenever he had been a patient, he was questioned and maybe tested by his colleagues. Then he was either directed to have more testing done or was given a prescription to alleviate his problem. "But with this approach," he said, "*you actually do something that changes the patient* and you see these immediate changes that result from your treatment. It's so basic—you treat someone to fix their body, you get it working better, you instruct them in healthy living, and you stimulate their nervous system in a way that improves their health and brings a sense of well-being. I'm just astounded."

He marveled that he had never learned so much or left an appointment actually feeling different, feeling so much better, and being immediately out of pain. He was even a bit remorseful that he had never done this for his own patients, but he didn't know where to begin. He could see how people might actually enjoy a visit with their doctor and was grateful to me for helping with his knee problem and his health and especially for introducing him to a whole new world of healthcare.

I reminded him of the different realms we operate in. As a mainstream doctor trained in the identification and treatment of disease, primarily acute disease, of course this holistic approach was a different experience for him.

Optimizing health, not alleviating symptoms

Tom noted that even if someone didn't have a specific symptom, functional testing could identify dysfunctions and lead to improved health. I acknowledged his open-mindedness and said to him what I say to other grateful patients, "Tell your friends."

I've learned in my treatment of healthy world-class and Olympic athletes that everyone has at least one weak link, no matter their level of development or performance. Most great athletes know what it is, and it often changes during their career. It could be a knee or shoulder problem, or a specific muscle problem, or their breathing or endurance. Whatever it is, when you improve the specific body function that created the weak link, your whole performance improves. It is a joy to witness the human spirit soaring to new levels of excellence and performance.

Most athletes who use this kind of holistic healthcare discover the innumerable benefits in working to optimize the function of all body parts. As their weak links get stronger, not only does their health improve, but so does their performance. They usually end up referring their friends and teammates, and everyone wonders why they didn't know about this before. As I said earlier, much of this is relatively new, and many people are just now hearing of it.

Tom and I had one other area to explore. It had to do with his negative attitude toward exercise, and I wanted to be sure he was not going to sabotage his progress.

An Emotional Alignment with Health

While Tom was enthusiastic about the improvements to his health and willing to change his diet, take supplements, and lessen his stress, the one recommendation he struggled with was exercise. He disliked his attitude and was apologetic, but he admitted to a mental block about it. His rational mind knew all the reasons why he should exercise, but he just didn't.

I appreciated his honesty. I also thought there was a way we could deal with his negative attitude. I look at all three sides of the triad of health—structural, chemical, and emotional—and work to get all three sides working together for the benefit of the patient. So far Tom and I had investigated and treated structurally and chemically, and we had made significant, measurable improvements in those areas. I was fairly sure our results would be enhanced if we addressed the emotional side of the triad.

Tom was hesitant. I assured him that it wouldn't interfere with anything we had done. But I told him we didn't have to do this right then or ever, for that matter. I left it up to him. After some hesitation and thought, he agreed, noting that everything we'd done so far had helped him.

I was curious to know if he'd had such a hesitation or internal resistance when he started taking an antidepressant.

"No, not really," he replied. He had just started taking the medication. But this seemed different—like he was going to have to perhaps face some major issue, not just take a pill.

I promised to make it as painless as possible and reassured him that he would not have to deal with anything in a major way, except for possibly his disbelief. And it was even OK if he didn't believe it; it would work anyway. It had to do with the circuitry in his nervous system.

He finally gave the go-ahead, still sounding a bit reluctant and clearly out of his comfort zone. He wondered why I thought there was some emotional thing affecting him.

I reminded him that he had told me several different ways that he hated exercise and that he even felt like he had a mental block about exercising. He told me how he used to love playing basketball, but that was different for him because it was a sport and it was fun to play. He made the distinction about exercise and described it as a chore that he just couldn't get himself to do, no matter how hard he tried.

He certainly wasn't the only person who didn't like exercise or who had trouble fitting it into a daily schedule. We needed to address his unwillingness, because aerobic exercise was so critical for Tom to help rebuild his adrenals and train his body to burn fat for more sustained energy and increased production of anti-inflammatory chemicals by his Inner Pharmacy. The benefits would be enormous. But it was unlikely I could say or tell him anything he didn't already know to convince him to start aerobic exercise and continue doing it, five times a week, forever.

Psychological reversal

What I did do, however was to test for a "psychological reversal." This involves observing how his body reacted to specific statements. First, I tested a muscle, his pectoralis major, to use as an indicator. As long as it tested strong, I knew it was on, or in other words, being facilitated by his nervous system. Then I instructed Tom to say a series of statements aloud, starting with "I want to be healthy."

I would then retest the muscle to see if it stayed on. If his brain and body were in synch and believed the statement to be true, the muscle would stay on.

After "I want to be healthy," the muscle stayed on. This was normal. Then I asked him to say, "I want to be sick." He was naturally quite hesitant, but I explained that he didn't need to believe it; it was just for this test.

After he said, "I want to be sick," I tested the pectoralis muscle. It tested weak, or shut off. Again, this was a normal result. The weakening showed that his body was not congruent with the thought of wanting to be sick.

Sometimes, people weaken from saying, "I want to be healthy," and stay strong from saying, "I want to be sick." That would be considered a massive psychological reversal about being healthy. Though they think their desire is to be healthy, the reversal actually works against their conscious attempts to be healthy. With this kind of reversal, they usually have several different health problems and never seem to get better. They also frequently and unknowingly do things to sabotage their health.

Tom contemplated the meaning of psychological reversal. Since he was congruent with the idea of wanting to be healthy, we went on to "I want to be happy."

After saying, "I want to be happy," Tom's pectoralis muscle stayed "on." I then asked him to say, "I want to be miserable." The muscle weakened, which was normal. He didn't have a psychological reversal about wanting to be healthy or happy. If he had been reversed on either of those, I would have corrected them before proceeding.

I next told him to say, "I want to exercise." He didn't believe it to be true, but he said it anyway. This time, the pectoralis muscle clearly shut off and tested very weak.

He was not a bit surprised and asked if this was like a lie detector. "Kind of," I said. "It does reveal the truth."

Whether the muscle is on or off relative to a stated idea lets us know what message the nervous system is communicating to the body. The message your body gets may or may not be what you consciously believe; what's more, you may even be unaware of the message. In terms of Tom's psychological reversal about wanting to exercise, he was aware of the result. Yet he didn't know how it was affecting him or how to get himself to exercise. His logical mind knew all the reasons why exercise would be good for him, but this reversal blocked him from doing what would be good for his body.

Many of us have reversals we are totally unaware of. We can be reversed about almost anything, and the reversal usually holds us back from progressing in life. Common reversals have to do with being successful, losing weight, stopping smoking, exercising regularly, eating healthful foods, having supportive relationships—and the list of possibilities goes on and on.

Tom recalled a patient, a man who was already taking several medications to control his blood pressure, cholesterol, anxiety, and heartburn. His joints were painful and inflamed, as if he had been running for weeks. He was exhausted, as if he had been chased by a tiger. Tom gave him another medication for his joint pain. But now, in hindsight, Tom believed that the patient's own brain was likely creating his symptoms, because it thought there was a tiger. He was realizing how often his treatments actually enabled people to keep running from their imaginary tigers.

Hans Selye's research on stress demonstrated that laboratory animals developed the same set of changes in their hormonal and immune systems when exposed to stress. These changes he termed the "triad of stress," which affects the adrenals and the immune and digestive systems.

Not only do our bodies respond to stress in predictable ways, but *our bodies actually respond to our perception of stress.* Two people can respond to the same stressful event in different physiological ways, depending on how they interpret it. One person could perceive a specific stress as a major threat and experience a dramatic fight-or-flight response of their sympathetic nervous system. Another person could perceive that same stressor as "no big deal" or "not worth getting upset over" and have no physical or emotional fight-or-flight response in their nervous system.

People often have all the symptoms of the fight-or-flight response, even when tigers aren't actually chasing them. Frequently, in chronic disease, there is no tiger! But if you think there is, your body will respond exactly the same as if there were a tiger in pursuit.

The point is that *our bodies respond to what is going on in the brain, not to what is going on in the environment.* The average person's physical response to a tennis ball approaching at a hundred miles an hour is a different response from that of a top-ranked tennis player. What one brain perceives as the attack of an object, another brain perceives as a routine opportunity to hit a tennis ball.

This all means that your body is responding to the messages it gets from your brain. How you view the world has a huge impact on the function of your body and on your aging process. In other words, your attitudes directly influence what goes on in your body.

That is why I was interested in correcting Tom's psychological reversal about wanting to exercise. The chances of him exercising regularly and getting benefits from it would be greatly enhanced if his body responded with strength, with muscles turning "on," not "off," when he *thought* about wanting to exercise.

So many of us want to change and improve our bodies or somehow change our lives. When you realize that your current life is a product of the messages you have sent out with your thoughts, you know that your thoughts and attitudes contain enormous power and potential for change. But even if you are sending good, constructive, healthy messages to your body and out to the world, the circuitry of your nervous system has to be working properly so that the correct message gets sent!

Tom had heard a lot about "mind-body medicine," and some of his medical colleagues even considered it to be a conventional approach. He recognized that just like everyone else, he was already creating his situation in life through his thoughts. It wasn't like he had never done that before, and now, all of a sudden, he was going to start creating his life. He had been doing it all along, and his current life was the result.

The psychological reversal is a glitch in circuitry, a defect that causes us to unknowingly create problems for ourselves. Correcting your psychological reversals allows your own mental efforts to create solutions rather than further problems.

Obviously, not everyone has been tested for psychological reversals, and it's likely some people don't have any. But most of us have one or more, commonly in the one or more areas of our lives that aren't working as well as we would like. We all know people who are very successful in many ways but who struggle with relationships or with their health. Others may be remarkably healthy but never attain the degrees of success or financial security they seem to deserve. Those people usually have reversals about success or wealth. I have seen competitive athletes who spent most of their careers coming in second or third only to later learn that they were reversed about winning.

Psychological reversals are common. Be suspicious of having a reversal in any area of your life in which your frequently struggle or in which results never seem to match the effort you expend toward them. That is a broad statement, but it is a good starting place if you are interested in the possibility of identifying a reversal.

The forward-bending test

Some people seem to be able to test themselves for a reversal, although results are more consistent and reliable with a qualified muscle tester doing the testing. For a self-test, Dr. Roger Callahan, a psychologist who wrote about psychological reversal in the early 1980s, suggested that people to do a "forward-bending" test. It can be done standing, although many people find it easier to do lying down.

I had Tom start by lying face up on the examining table. Then I asked him to sit up and simply bend forward, keeping his knees straight and locked, and try to touch his toes, without bouncing or reaching beyond what was comfortable. He could reach only part way down his shins to a few inches above his ankles, and he commented that he had never been very flexible. I told him to do it a few times to loosen up, and then I would mark where his fingertips reached on his shins.

After Tom stretched forward a few times, I made a pen mark on his shins where his fingertips touched. The marks would serve as a baseline to monitor for a potential change. Then he lay back down, and I explained that he would next say aloud the same statements he had said earlier, and then, after each, test the forward bending.

Tom began, saying, "I want to be healthy," and then bending forward again, he was surprised to see that he reached about a half inch beyond the baseline marks on his shins. It could be he was loosening up more, but it was also possible we were seeing a change.

He lay back down, and I asked him to say, "I want to be sick," and then bend again. This time he could not bend as far forward, no matter how hard he tried. His fingertips were almost an inch short of the line. His body, his neuromusculoskeletal system, changed a full inch and a half in its ability to bend, based on what he said and whether he was congruent with it.

Self-testing doesn't always provide such definitive results and doesn't work on everyone, but it appeared to be working on him. It agreed with the findings of the earlier muscle testing. The neurological facilitation and inhibition that had turned on and off his shoulder muscle also affected many other muscles in the body. The forward bending is a crude, composite test of a number of muscles.

The fact that Tom reached farther with "I want to be healthy" implies that he was congruent with that statement and incongruent with "I want to be sick," the statement that limited his ability to bend forward. On the contrary, if he had reached farther with "I want to be sick," it would imply he was more in agreement with wanting to be sick. That would represent a psychological reversal about health, of which he might be unconscious. If he were reversed about health, he might have chronic health problems that don't respond to the usual treatment, and he may even notice himself unconsciously doing things to sabotage his health.

To test his response to the exercise issue, Tom said, "I want to exercise," and then bent forward. He could reach only about one inch short of the baseline marks. Then I asked him to say, "I hate exercise." He laughed as he enthusiastically said this one. We both laughed as he bent forward a full inch past the ink marks. Yes, the latter was a true statement, and it would remain true as long as he was reversed about wanting to exercise.

Tom said he was ready to make a change. He really did want to be healthy, and he wouldn't mind exercising if he could just get himself to do it regularly. He didn't claim he would enjoy it, but he would do what was required, and he really wanted me to correct his reversal if I could.

Correcting the reversal

There are several ways to correct a reversal, but to keep it simple, I did a basic correction that Dr. Callahan developed in 1981.[4] It involves tapping on specific acupuncture points on the hand while a person says the statement that weakened him and which he wants to get congruent with. In Tom's case the statement was, "I want to exercise." Stimulating the acupuncture points while the statement is spoken in effect resets the circuitry. The result is that the person's mind-body complex becomes congruent with the statement being spoken.

Could this technique be used to get someone congruent with a statement with dangerous or unethical ramifications? No, it doesn't work that way. Based as it is on the wisdom of the body, correcting a reversal simply involves resetting the body's circuitry with natural, life-supporting, positive statements that advance health and personal development. Resetting the body to its natural state of health and truth is different from creating a new, unnatural, negative, or devious condition.

Since the person with the reversal says the statement during the tapping, if a statement didn't feel or sound right to him, he shouldn't engage in the procedure. I also reminded Tom that I had asked for his permission before pursuing this, which is a wise and respectful policy before doing any emotional testing and treatment.

Traditional Chinese medicine has used acupuncture points for the past few thousand years. Acupuncture is a phenomenal world of diagnosis, treatment, and restoration of the body to health and balance with nature. When people ask if acupuncture really works, I like to answer, "What exists persists." There is simply no way that acupuncture would still be around after thousands of years and widely used by perhaps a billion people if it were not effective.

Acupuncture meridians and points have been measured electrically, and not only do they exist, but they can be influenced in numerous ways. For example, in the treatment of psychological reversals, tapping on the acupuncture point is more effective than inserting an acupuncture needle, presumably because the tapping itself influences the nervous system as well as the acupuncture point being tapped on.

The particular acupuncture point we were going to tap on is located on the small-intestine meridian. There are energy channels, called meridians, that correlate with the major organs and functions in the body. The small-intestine meridian doesn't physically go over the small intestine. It starts on the little finger of each hand, travels up the arm, over the shoulder and neck, and ends on the face, just in front of the ear. Measurable electromagnetic energy travels up the meridian. Each of the nineteen specific acupuncture points on the small-intestine meridian is like a mini-resistor in the circuit. If stimulated, each point can affect certain functions in the body, primarily related to the role of the small intestine. Each point also affects the physical area where that point is located, which is why acupuncturists may stimulate them to help a neck, shoulder, or arm problem. As seen in figure 6, the primary point that corrects psychological reversals is a small-intestine-related point located on the outer edge of the hand, just below the base of the little finger.

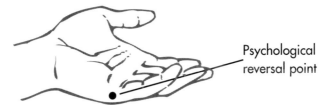

Psychological
reversal point

Figure 6

I would tap for about thirty seconds on this acupuncture point on each of Tom's hands while he said aloud and repeatedly, "I want to exercise regularly." Then he himself continued tapping the edges of both hands against each other while he said the statement.

After a minute of tapping and repeating his statement, Tom made an interesting observation. He said it had felt funny at first to say that statement. And he didn't think it was because he was self-conscious. There had been a resistance or an emotional charge in saying it, but now with the tapping, it felt much easier. I could hear a distinct difference in his voice versus how it had sounded before the tapping.

Before, it had been timid, hesitant, disbelieving. With the tapping, it sounded confident, like he meant it.

What we had just done was a basic correction. To test it, I told him to say, without tapping, "I want to exercise regularly." He firmly stated it, and I then retested his pectoralis muscle, finding that it tested very strong, clearly was on, and stayed that way when Tom affirmed that he wanted to exercise regularly.

We also retested his forward bending as another way to measure his body's response. He said the statement again and bent forward over an inch past the baseline marks. So now, saying that he wants to exercise actually gave him more strength and balance than before the tapping. I see this kind of amazing change on a daily basis.

To reinforce his new healthy attitude toward exercise, I instructed him to tap the edges of his hands together while saying the statement for at least thirty seconds, three times a day for the next few weeks. I also recommended low-impact exercise, such as cycling or swimming, which was unlikely to aggravate his knee. He was to keep his left ankle taped until he got the orthotics and to focus on aerobic exercise, for now, at least five times a week. Using the heart-rate formula, we calculated his ideal aerobic heart rate. With the warm-up and cool-down, Tom would reap huge benefits from as little as thirty minutes a day. See chapter 7 for how to calculate the rate.

I recommended he make a thirty-minute appointment with himself for that afternoon and get started. The exercise would get his Inner Pharmacy producing more good chemicals, which would stimulate the healing process and support the positive changes we were making. I gave clear instructions that if he found himself resisting or avoiding the exercise, he was to do more frequent tapping, like once an hour if necessary.

Reversals for specific problems

Tom was ready. Yet there was one other potential psychological reversal we should address. If he had it, fixing it would be the frosting on the cake.

When Tom had said, "I want to be healthy," he meant it. He was not reversed. But had he been, that would have been what I call a "massive" reversal, because this very general statement affects the body in many different ways. It can be useful to test more specific statements within the broad category of health, such as, "I want to be totally healthy and 100 percent free of pain."

To evaluate for this possible reversal, Tom said this statement and I retested the pectoralis muscle, finding that it stayed "on." If he had weakened from that one, I would have done additional corrections on his body and then had him follow up with tapping while saying that specific phrase.

A variation is a statement about a specific body part a person has been struggling with, so I told Tom to say, "I want my left knee to be totally healthy and free of pain."

After saying this, his pectoralis muscle dramatically shut off. This weakening baffled Tom, who wondered if that meant he actually didn't want his knee to be totally healthy and free of pain.

It didn't mean he didn't want a healthy knee, but psychological reversals are quite uncanny. Tom may consciously want his knee to be healthy and free of pain, but somewhere in his system the circuitry had it jumbled up. His brain may have been generating the message for a healthy knee, but the message received by his knee or body could be just the opposite. Some communication problem within his circuitry was altering the message.

It could be as simple as the brain sends one message and the body receives another. But that is only a small piece of it. I believe there's a lot more to it.

Candace Pert, the discoverer of neuropeptide receptors on white blood cells, has contributed greatly to our understanding of the interconnectedness of mind and body. Using terminology that unifies the body and brain, she coined the term *psychosomatic communication network*.[5]

Though we don't fully understand the communication networks, the circuitry can be influenced, modified, and often corrected through procedures such as tapping acupuncture points.

So Tom corrected the specific knee reversal by tapping the edges of his hands together while saying repeatedly for thirty seconds, "I want my left knee to be totally healthy and free of pain."

After the tapping, his pectoralis muscle tested strong, staying on following the statement, "I want my left knee to be totally healthy and free of pain."

I was happy with his response and instructed him to add this tapping three times a day, along with the exercise phrase, for the next few weeks. His daily tapping would help to reprogram his system to be congruent with both these phrases, which should eventually become permanent.

The origin of psychological reversals

Where do psychological reversals come from and what causes them? As a doctor, Tom wanted some answers. I don't profess to know the answer. We in the scientific community don't totally know yet. Answers may come when we better understand more of the interconnectedness in the body. But one fascinating fact has to do with the small intestine. Correcting psychological reversal can be done by tapping on a specific acupuncture point located on the small-intestine meridian. This means that psychological reversals are significantly related to the small intestine, which has some very specific implications, one of which is that a problem in the small intestine could generate the communication error that becomes the reversal.

The vagus nerve, or the tenth cranial nerve, is the parasympathetic nerve that stimulates the stomach, heart, lungs, and other internal organs, including the intestines. The traditional view is that the vagus nerve carries messages from the brain to these organs. The vagus nerve helps to stimulate peristalsis, which keeps the intestines moving. Stress exacerbates gastrointestinal disorders, and frightening emotions can trigger spasms in the gut. Those examples probably represent messages being sent from the brain to the gut via the vagus nerve.

But in the early 1990s, researchers found that the vagus nerve also carries immune signals *from* the intestines *to* the brain.[6] We speak of our gut feelings and gut reactions, and there is physiological truth behind these phrases. Since the gut sends messages to the brain, we suspect that this circuitry is probably what is influenced when we tap the small-intestine point on the hand while saying the statement the body has reversed. In essence, a malfunction in the small intestine could lead to a psychological reversal, and this an example of the connection between the chemical and emotional sides of the triad of health.

Food allergies can create psychological reversals. In chapter 4, John's shoulder problem was created by his sensitivity to wheat. Food sensitivities commonly create problems in the gut. They can also cause people to have panic attacks or to become irritable and fatigued. The food triggers an adverse reaction within the immune system, producing an inflammatory response, the location of which varies according to the individual's genetic makeup. Some people are prone to reactions in the small intestine, and their emotions are then affected. Most of us have the concept that food allergies or sensitivities create only physical symptoms, but foods can just as easily affect our moods and our circuitry. "Comfort foods" give just that; is it any wonder that other foods can do just the opposite?

If Tom had a recurrence of his psychological reversals, one of the first additional tests I would recommend would be for a potential food sensitivity. The intestines are not merely devoted to digestion. The intestinal tract is also an immune-system organ, and it is the site of nearly two-thirds of the body's defense system.[7] A malfunction within this system can manifest in many different ways, ranging from malabsorption and subsequent nutrient deficiencies to immune, inflammatory, and even emotional problems. A bacterial imbalance in the intestines, frequently in the form of too many bad bacteria and not enough good bacteria, can disrupt the circuitry and lead to psychological reversals. Inflammatory gut problems are also commonly caused by medications, especially NSAIDs. Damage to the gastrointestinal system is an unfortunate and costly side effect of NSAIDs for many people, who ironically use these medications to control inflammation. To reiterate, anything that has an adverse effect on the small intestine could create a psychological reversal.

Because of the chemical-emotional connection, poor-quality diets—those loaded with sugar, bad fats, and artificial ingredients—can cause chemical and hormonal imbalances that may be a factor in the development of deviant or violent behavior.

Besides various intestinal problems, psychological reversals can also be caused by emotional trauma and the negative programming people receive while growing up. Tom may have had negative experiences or associations with exercise going back to his childhood. He may have heard people whine about how unpleasant exercise was for them and how much they hated it. A negative association could have come from some experience that he wasn't even conscious of or doesn't remember.

In addition to the testing I did on Tom, a more involved and detailed approach is the Neuro-Emotional Technique (NET). NET uses diagnostic muscle testing to evaluate the body's response to specific questions, allowing the practitioner to gather more information about the origin of the reversal. Once the origin is identified, specific treatments affecting the nervous-system circuitry disconnect the influence of a trauma or negative programming. With Tom, this could have been the next step, but there was a good chance he would maintain the correction if he did the routine tapping for a few weeks as instructed and maintained a good diet and exercise regimen.

While Tom was amazed at how I addressed his knee, which took me to his pelvis, foot, muscles, cranium, adrenal glands, and elsewhere, he really understood holistic healthcare through the psychological reversal. Instead of simply telling him what to do, holistic care makes a change in the patient, reinforcing healthy behavior by making the patient congruent with it.

Addressing your potential reversals can make lifestyle changes easier, especially if you struggle with your diet and exercise and attitudes. Telling yourself to exercise and eat healthfully, or hearing it from your doctor, doesn't often work. I think that's why so many of my colleagues in mainstream medicine give up on trying to change patients' lifestyles. Instead, Western medical practitioners focus on medications that will at least control symptoms and keep the patient out of immediate danger, while all the while the patient continues an unhealthy lifestyle.

Historically and chronologically, the original credit for this work goes to the founder of Applied Kinesiology, Dr. George Goodheart, the brilliant chiropractor who, in 1964, discovered the value of using manual muscle testing as a way to measure body function.

In the 1970s, Dr. John Diamond, an M.D. psychiatrist, used muscle testing in the emotional arena and made enormous contributions in testing for emotional patterns and connecting them with the acupuncture energy in the body.

In the 1980s, Dr. Roger Callahan, a psychologist, named psychological reversal and developed ways to correct it. He also obtained phenomenal results by applying his techniques to the treatment of phobias. Also in the 1980s, Dr. Scott Walker, a chiropractor, discovered and developed the Neuro-Emotional Technique (NET). In addition to helping in the treatment of many health problems, NET is very effective in the arena of human performance, helping people to exceed their previous limitations in all areas of their lives.

The teachings and systems developed by each of these innovators have since branched out and are now used by thousands of doctors for the benefit of millions of patients. The chiropractors, who utilize the emotional procedures from Applied Kinesiology and NET, are able to combine the emotional work with corrections to the spine, which allows them to efficiently reset the nervous system to assist the correction of the communication error that has become a psychological reversal. It lends itself very nicely to treating people who are "stuck" or somehow blocked in the pursuit of their goals or the improvement of their health and wellness.

Many psychologists now use these procedures, finding that they can *powerfully change the patient* who is engaged in psychotherapy. Dr. Diamond's work grew into the field of Behavioral Kinesiology. Dr. Callahan's techniques grew into Thought Field Therapy (TFT), and a dynamic offshoot became known as Emotional Freedom Techniques (EFT). Many in the exciting and emerging field of Energy Psychology use these procedures as a major component of their professional practices.

Tom's depression

Our discussion of the emotional side of the triad of health prompted another question from Tom, who wondered if I thought this holistic approach could have helped with his depression, for which he had been taking antidepressant medication for years.

I reflected on what he had told me earlier about his depression—that it came on after his knee injury and seemed related to no longer being able to play basketball. He had also been under a lot of stress from medical school, was becoming less and less physically active, and had felt the effects of aging, even at a young age.

If he had been treated structurally, chemically, and emotionally back then, he probably could have avoided a lot of problems and some major accelerated aging.

Structurally, if someone had corrected his ankle, knee, and pelvic misalignments and the shut-off muscles that were not supporting his knee, he probably could have returned to playing sports shortly after the injury. Since playing basketball had a major stress-reducing effect for him and kept him physically active, he may not have even developed the depression. He could have avoided years of taking an antidepressant and the years of NSAID damage to his gastrointestinal tract. Hindsight is twenty-twenty, but these are reasonable possibilities if he had received good structural treatment after the injuries to his ankle and knee.

Chemically, if his knee problem twenty years earlier had been evaluated holistically, the adrenal component would have likely been identified, due to the adrenal-related muscles that were shut off and not supporting the knee. In the course of treating his fatigued adrenal glands, the chemical imbalance that later contributed to his depression might have been addressed. Treating his body's response to stress back then, especially with cranial treatment, would also have turned the normal stomach-enzyme production back on, so he could have digested proteins and not developed the protein deficiency that contributed to the joint-surface deterioration of the injured knee and added to the depression. There may have been several chemical components to his depression, which could have been treated naturally.

On the *emotional* side, it was difficult to say. Depressed people often have a massive psychological reversal about wanting to be happy or healthy. He may have had an imbalance in his acupuncture energy that could have contributed to the depression. Functional testing or a good acupuncturist could have identified that, twenty years earlier, if he had seen a practitioner who evaluates for and treats dysfunction.

While I am no fan of antidepressants, I am definitely not a fan of people going around in states of depression. It's dangerous, unpleasant, and for most depressed people, nonproductive. Having said that, I emphasize the value of *treating the patient who has the depression.* Medications, when used successfully, can restore a lost quality of life to a depressed person. But certainly, using them indefinitely on every depressed person, without looking for the cause of their depression, is questionable. Medications are one way to deal with a chemical imbalance in the body. So is correcting an abnormal physiology, allowing the body to heal itself and function normally.

A disturbing trend in technologized nations is the increased use of antidepressants in children. Perhaps many children taking antidepressants are receiving the best and most appropriate treatment. But many could be helped even more by improving their diets and nutritional status and their chemical and glandular imbalances; beginning exercise and stress-reduction programs; eliminating food sensitivities; restoring balance to their nervous systems through spinal and cranial corrections; and addressing their psychological reversals.

For chronic symptoms, correcting the underlying problem is usually the safest and the most effective and direct route to obtaining the desired result, and it often corrects other problems as well. Take, for example, someone who is chronically sick, succumbing to frequent, even serial, infections, and who is almost constantly on antibiotics. The natural healthcare approach would evaluate the function of their immune system, particularly the thymus gland, which helps the body to fight infections. In this scenario, the thymus is usually found to be underactive, and as a holistic practitioner, I would treat the patient in ways that normalize the thymus with various reflexes and acupuncture points, and then I would have the patient take specific vitamins and herbs to stimulate and rebuild the thymus gland.

The direct result is often an improved immune-system function, which means less frequent and less severe infections. The additional benefit is that the patient often feels much better emotionally. And it's not just because she is no longer sick all the time. It is quite interesting that the medical definition for a malfunctioning thymus gland, dysthymia, is chronic discontent. When the thymus functions better, not only does the immune system function more effectively, but people actually experience contentment.

The common condition of a subclinical low thyroid function causes people to exhibit symptoms such as fatigue, depression, thinning hair, or an inability to lose weight. It can be very difficult to get them to exercise, since people with low thyroids are often lethargic and tend to be unmotivated. It is quite amazing how much a person's outlook and even their motivation can be affected by their glandular function. The very thing, the low thyroid, that contributed to the weight problem also made them unmotivated to exercise or take other actions to change their situation. In this example, improving thyroid function could be the key to improving health as well as correcting an array of emotional difficulties. Looking at it holistically entails the constant challenge of seeing it from a bigger perspective, but doing so allows one to see many truly amazing overlaps and interconnections.

Summary

For active people, injuries are inevitable. *It's how you take care of them* that determines how well your injuries heal. In this era of saber-toothed tigers lurking all around us, it's inevitable to develop imbalance and distortions in the autonomic nervous, glandular, and immune systems. Dealing with and correcting the imbalance is much more direct and efficient than adding one medication after another to modify the symptoms caused by the imbalance.

It's all about health and healthy aging, and it's really quite simple. We could boil it down to three things. First of all, you need a properly functioning body. That's where healthcare comes in—to correct and reset your body after injuries, traumas, and stresses, and to keep it balanced to withstand the challenges of life.

Second, you need to give your body good raw materials in the form of diet and nutritional supplements. One could even argue that positive emotional stimulation and support could fit into this category. But, just to keep it simple, let's emphasize the chemical building blocks that the body's Inner Pharmacy uses to make good chemicals.

Third, you need activity, both physical and mental, to stimulate the Inner Pharmacy to convert the raw materials into good chemicals. Aerobic exercise favors the breakdown of fats into the production of energy and the body's own anti-inflammatory chemicals. Stress-reducing activities are critical to shift the Inner Pharmacy away from the overproduction of stress hormones and toward the production of non-stress hormones. Activity, in the form of any movement, deep breathing, and physical exercise, is critical to stimulate and maintain life.

Within this third category of activity exists a psychological component that may be more spiritual than physical. We'll call it intention, and it includes the desire to be healthy and whole. Keeping in mind how the doctor's reversal held him back, you can see that it is not only important to have healthy beliefs, but it is also important to be congruent with those beliefs. If you are psychologically reversed, your very desire to be healthy could be having the opposite effect on your body.

This is a simple approach to health and wholeness, and it is what happens naturally when we don't get in the way. When babies come into this world, they innately do these three things quite well. Even with their own unique genetics and varying degrees of limitations, their new bodies usually work pretty well. They have a totally natural and inherent desire to be active, to eat foods that are good for their bodies, and to play.

Somewhere along the line, however, the damage starts. They take a few falls and become injured. They are presented with highly sugared and artificial foods that alter their tastes. They encounter negative attitudes and become programmed to think in limited ways. They become sedentary, watching far too much television, and their active lifestyles are further dampened by the influence of inactive parents and schools that don't see the value in physical education.

Buckminster Fuller, the revolutionary thinker and doer who transformed our concept of our "spaceship earth," said it very well. Later in his astonishing career, he was asked how he possibly accomplished so much more in his lifetime than other children who grew up in the same era. His simple reply was, "I was less damaged than most."

Perhaps that sums it up best. Our country and our economy are being crippled by people who are continuing to be damaged and don't know that options exist other than trying to cover up the damage. The epidemic of chronic disease is not being addressed by covering up the symptoms. It's time to undo the damage and create an epidemic of health.

Part 3, "Health Planning 101," will guide you in creating your own healthy lifestyle, one that uses these three things to enable your Inner Pharmacy to create health and quality time.

Part 3

Health Planning 101

6

IT'S ABOUT TIME:
CREATE YOUR HEALTHY LIFESTYLE

Many parts of this section might seem rather basic. As a matter of fact, at some point in your life, most likely as a youngster, you knew much of what follows. Somewhere along the line, you got busy and may have stopped doing the basics that could keep you healthy and balanced throughout life. You may have developed health problems, some of which advanced into chronic disease. And perhaps you haven't realized that you can take charge of your health and massively improve it. The normal response to a busy life is to just keep running forward, blinders on, without giving much attention to where we're running. We're going to start by removing the blinders.

How to Create Time

Time is one of the great mysteries of life. As you get older, time passes faster and there seems to be less of it. Time becomes more precious, yet many of us lose respect for it. We spend all our time—without investing any of it to create time for later in our lives. Most of us try to save money for retirement and special things, but we don't even think of saving time for later.

You really can create quality time for yourself. Creating time may sound like something out of a science-fiction movie, but it's not complicated. As a matter of fact, it is straightforward. It's simply a matter of doing certain things on a regular basis. It is so simple that following the easy steps described in the next two chapters will almost guarantee you more quality time, now and for years to come.

I say *almost* guarantee, because stuff happens. Accidents and illnesses affect people and seem to be unavoidable, at least based on what we currently know. So we just do our best to improve our lives, knowing we may not be able to control all the factors that affect the future. Many people give up on trying to improve their health because they think they'll probably get some bad disease or die in an accident and just lose it all anyway. Sure, unpredictable things happen, but it's much more common for predicable ones to happen. If it turns out that you do have a future, it's much better if you have prepared for it. In the case of middle-aged people, doing the right things to prepare for the future is critical in determining if we even have one. I like to say, "*Health happens.*" It happens, that is, as long as you do certain things to take care of your health, help it along, and ensure that it grows.

Most likely, when you were ten, you rarely had to think about your health. You probably had the opportunity of being able to take it for granted. You may have gotten sick once in a while or were influenced by someone else's illness, but that was about the only time you ever had to think about health.

Contrast your relationship to health, as a ten-year-old, with your current situation or perhaps a time later in life when something in your body was hurting constantly. What if your stomach or knee or back or shoulder hurt all the time? Or what if you were always tired and never felt like doing anything? Or what if doing almost anything made you feel miserable because it hurt so much and took so much energy?

This kind of debilitation may very well happen eventually. Even so, what if you could put it off, delay it, postpone it for ten or twenty years? What if you could actually feel good for an extra ten or twenty or even more years?

Of course you want that. Everyone does, yet it somehow doesn't seem so obvious to a lot of people. They don't know what to do and how to do it so they can have these years of feeling good. That's why it is so important to respect health and to see its value. We run our-selves ragged trying to make more money, and we forget that money has little value if you don't feel good. We've gotten so accustomed to reacting to disease that we really have to adjust our thinking to real-ize that it is much better to create health.

For most people, living a healthy lifestyle is more a motivational challenge than an informational one. You already know that a healthy diet and regular exercise both contribute to health. I'm not going to give you more information on that, but rather, I want to try to shift your perspective.

First, let's briefly revisit the lifestyle syndrome in which dysfunc-tion in the body precedes chronic disease, which is so fundamental to understanding the distinction between treating disease and creating health. This overlooked distinction contains the essence of why health problems are spiraling out of control and the mainstream medical system cannot solve the problem. At the core of the problem are deeply ingrained societal attitudes and cultural factors that create lifestyles out of synch with our genetic makeup. These unhealthy lifestyles accelerate the aging process by altering the physiology of how our bodies function. The altered physiology and dysfunction in the body create ongoing symptoms, which then become labeled as chronic disease. As it progresses, it creates more severe symptoms, requiring more medications. Never is the cause of the altered physi-ology that created the symptoms in the first place addressed.

It is not the fault of traditional Western medicine that we have this problem. Yet a traditional "this-for-that" approach is unlikely to solve the healthcare crisis. The billions of dollars poured into high-technology diagnosis help advance our understanding of the body. The billions spent on pharmaceutical development and use may help people live longer and better tolerate their chronic conditions. But these medications usually have to be taken forever, rarely address the cause of the problems, and frequently create side effects that trade one problem for another. Furthermore, by easing some of the trouble-some symptoms of chronic disease, expensive medications lure us into thinking we are doing everything possible to treat the disease. In fact, the medications are treating symptoms and missing the opportunity to interrupt the advancement of the condition itself. And most important, the spending of all these billions pales in comparison to the effect of a mass of people simply creating more healthy lifestyles and living them on a daily basis. We can slow the aging process, extend our lives, and delay the onset of many chronic, degenerative conditions. Yes, there is a way to create quality time. And creating health will enormously decrease your need to treat disease.

So, to create a healthy lifestyle for yourself and your family, the first step is to create your own health plan. The next step is living your plan.

Plan for Health

How would you respond to the question, "Do you have a health plan?"

Perhaps you have never considered it before or are wondering what one is. Here is another question: "Do you have a financial plan?"

Like many Americans, you do. We have been drilled into planning financially for our future. But planning for your health is just as important. It's about time—time you can add to your years.

Get a paper and pen. At the top of the sheet, write "My Health Plan." Then a bit lower, write "Where I Am" and write down your age and your current state of health, classifying it as excellent, good, mediocre, or poor. If you have not had any recent professional assessment of your health, I strongly encourage you to do that soon.

Next, make a table with two headings: "Health Assets" and "Health Liabilities." List at least five of each. Assets might include a strong genetic constitution, if your siblings, parents, or grandparents lived into their eighties or nineties. Other assets might be that you maintain your ideal weight, that you like to exercise and enjoy physical recreation, that you naturally hover toward a healthy diet, or perhaps that you have periodic medical checkups and follow a regular approach to early detection and to prevention.

Liabilities can come from the genes you inherited, such as a family history of heart disease, diabetes, cancer, or arthritis. Other liabilities are if you are overweight or addicted to sugar, bad fats, or fast foods. Also in the liability column would be a sedentary job, an aversion to exercise, or ongoing or frequent stress. Old injuries should be listed as well as anything that prevents you from being more physically active or from following a healthful diet. Problems with your digestive system, frequent episodes of back pain or headaches, frequent illness or fatigue, or current medical conditions all go in this column.

Now write "Where I Want to Be." For the immediate and distant future, write down your goals for retirement, recreation, family, work, and so on. Under that, to represent the state of health you want, make three columns: "Age 65," "Age 75," and "Age 85." Under each, write down a specific goal as an example of what you want to be able to do at each of those ages. You might want to write down the calendar year that corresponds with each of those ages. You may also want to calculate the ages of your children and speculate on the ages of your potential grandchildren and even great-grandchildren as you reach these landmarks. It really helps if you have an emotional word-picture as your goal for each of those years. As with all goal-setting, have high expectations of yourself. Aim high. Don't settle for a sedentary life of watching the world go by until you are ready for that stage.

Now you have a sense of where you are and where you want to go. So what will you do to get there? Write down "How to Get There." Addressing this question involves growing your assets and minimizing or eliminating your liabilities. Tools that can help you to do this are covered in chapter 7, "Getting It Right," and you will probably want to complete your plan after reading that chapter. Be assured that you don't have to do this all yourself. You create and implement your plan. Other health professionals and resources assist you along the way. In that chapter, you will discover various health-promoting activities to engage in regularly.

Creating a healthy lifestyle usually requires the discipline to break some old habits and establish some new ones. Since many of us claim we don't have time to exercise, to eat properly, or to take care of ourselves, be sure you address this time issue. The other frequent excuse is that exercise takes too much energy and leaves you depleted when you were already exhausted to begin with. This misconception, along with the possibility of injuring or aggravating an existing problem, is addressed in the next chapter. If you do exercise correctly, you will have much more energy, clarity, and productivity, and you will be in a better frame of mind as you meet the challenges of each day.

It's about Time

So let's discuss the time issue. If you're being chased by a saber-toothed tiger, of course, it's difficult to plan for and think rationally about the future. The immediate crisis not only changes your perception of time, but it alters the value you place on time twenty years in the future. To varying degrees, we are all in that situation, and it creates a shortsighted focus on the present. Hence, part of your challenge is to slow down. Stop right now for a few moments. Even though you are sitting relatively still, your mind may be racing about your deadlines and commitments. Just sit still and take a few deep breaths to slow your mind and clear your head.

What you want to do is develop a realistic awareness of where your time goes and how you can use some of it to create a future. Time is like money: the biggest reason people don't save and invest money for the future is that many of us spend all that we earn—and sometimes more. If you don't save money because you have no money left over to save, the solution is simply to not spend all that you earn. One way to do that is to pay yourself first. That means to take at least 10 percent of what you earn each month and set it aside. Save it. Invest it. Pay yourself that 10 percent first, and then pay your bills and spend the rest as you choose. The 10 percent accumulates and multiplies into a substantial savings that can bring security and opportunity later in life, as long as you maintain your health so you can enjoy it.

Let's apply this same principle to health planning. You can create health and quality time for your future by investing time now. Simply invest 10 percent of your leisure time each week into health-promoting activities. The time you invest will improve your health, decrease your medical expenses, and enormously improve your chances of having a future to enjoy. You will be increasing your health assets and decreasing your liabilities.

You may wonder what 10 percent of your leisure time amounts to and how you would be able to carve out that amount of time from your busy schedule. It's simple. Let's do some basic calculations.

There are 168 hours in a week. We'll consider the average work week to be forty hours and add another five hours a week for commuting, totaling forty-five hours. (And even commuting can be health-promoting: read or listen to material about health.)

Eight hours of sleep a night totals another fifty-six hours for the week. Using conservative figures for eating three healthy meals a day—say a half hour for breakfast, a half hour for lunch, and an hour for dinner—makes two hours a day, or another fourteen hours a week. Time spent on bathing and hygiene varies, but say roughly three hours a week.

With these estimates, that leaves fifty hours a week of "leisure time." Now, "leisure time" may not be the most accurate description, especially if you are raising children or have other time-consuming obligations, but you get the idea. The point is, the averages provide you with fifty available hours each week. And 10 percent of fifty is five hours a week to invest in your health. Just imagine the dividends you could receive from simply investing five hours a week into improving your health!

If you think it would be impossible to come up with five hours a week to invest in your health, I suggest that first you take a close look at where your time currently goes. Most of us have black holes where time mysteriously disappears, the most common of which is the television. Second, consider the high cost to you if you don't invest time in health-promoting activities. The downward spiral of unhealthy aging takes a huge toll on your productivity and quality of life as well as increasing the deterioration and dysfunction that leads to chronic disease and its high costs.

To find those five hours, I strongly suggest you simply make the decision to pay yourself first. *Don't spend all your time* without first setting aside at least 10 percent of it for yourself. If you are so consumed by taking care of other people and causes, consider what airlines tell us to do in the event of a loss of air pressure in a plane. They tell us to put on our own oxygen mask before assisting others. Airlines know that if you don't take care of yourself first, you may be totally useless to others, no matter how much you love them. Likewise, investing 10 percent of your leisure time is far from being selfish. On the contrary, it may greatly increase your ability to help others and prevent them from having to take care of *you* prematurely.

You probably use some form of time-management system, such as a calendar, day-timer, or PDA to organize your days, weeks, and months, which means it is simply a matter of scheduling five hours a week for *you*. Schedule the five hours just as you would schedule any other high-priority appointment. Enter the appointment and then keep it. In chapter 7 are health-promoting ways you can use your five hours. But for now, it is simply a matter of doing it: start the investment in your health right now by making a commitment to invest at least five hours every week in health-promoting activities. At the bottom of your health plan, write, "I commit to invest five hours each week in activities that will promote my health." Sign your name under this statement and date it.

You now have the core ingredients of a health plan: (1) a list of your health assets and liabilities; (2) your goals that represent the state of health you want to possess at ages sixty-five, seventy-five, and eighty-five; and (3) your own commitment to invest 10 percent of your weekly leisure time into activities that will increase your health assets, decrease your liabilities, and help you to attain your goals for later in life.

Remember that healthy aging is an endurance event. You don't have to be perfect every step of the way, but it is essential that you establish and maintain healthy habits. If you get distracted and find yourself on a detour, just get back on track with your program. This whole process is fun. It is not a chore or any kind of torture or punishment.

You can even do some self-evaluation to make sure you do not have any psychological reversals that could sabotage your efforts. The simple test that follows will be accurate for most people, and I think you'll find it interesting. You can use the forward-bending test that I did with Tom in chapter 5. It's easier to do this test lying down, but if you don't have room, do the standing version. To loosen up, bend forward and try to touch your toes while keeping your knees straight. Do this a few times. You may be able to touch your toes or only reach part way down your shins. Regardless of how far you reach, that point will be a baseline for the test. After loosening up, repeat the forward bend, this time putting a dot on your shin or toes—wherever you reached. This is your baseline.

Now say aloud, "I want to be healthy." Then bend forward again and see if your forward bending reaches the same point or beyond. For comparison, say, "I want to be sick," and bend forward again. The difference that you may be seeing is based on how neuromuscular factors change when you think and say specific things. If you are able to bend farther forward, it is because of improved muscle balance in your body. If your forward bending is reduced or limited, it is because the muscles have tightened up and are more out of balance.

Approximately 75 percent will see a change in their forward bending after saying either statement. The other 25 percent will see no change following either statement. Don't feel badly if you didn't see a change. It's as if the computer in your nervous system doesn't have a particular program running at this time. Occasionally, the change in forward bending produces the same response from both statements, like bending farther or not as far following both statements, which means your program may not be working properly. Healthcare practitioners who use kinesiological techniques such as Applied Kinesiology and Neuro-Emotional Technique can do specific corrections on your body to activate and correct that program, which could be quite valuable for you.

If you did see a change, chances are that you bent farther forward after saying, "I want to be healthy," and not as far after saying, "I want to be sick." This response means you are congruent with wanting to be healthy and incongruent with wanting to be sick.

The opposite is true if you bent farther following "I want to be sick" and not as far following "I want to be healthy." This does not mean you want to be sick and don't want to be healthy. It really means that something has gotten jumbled up in the circuitry of your nervous system—a psychological reversal. A reversal can sabotage your attempts to improve your health. The 10 percent of the population who have this massive reversal about health have a much greater challenge in establishing and following a health plan than the other 90 percent who are congruent with wanting to be healthy. This 10 percent is not doomed to fail, but they have to work much harder to succeed.

Figure 6 on page 157 shows the acupuncture points on the edge of the hands, near the base of the little finger. If you have a reversal about health, tap your hands repeatedly together so these points meet each other, for about thirty seconds, while repeating, "I want to be healthy." It works if you say the phrase silently, but it works better if you say it aloud.

If you had the reversal and did the tapping, you can now retest yourself with the forward bending. Bend forward a few times to establish your baseline, which may have changed. Now say, "I want to be healthy," and bend forward again. Then say, "I want to be sick," and bend forward again. You should now see a whole different response from your body. Again, attaining and maintaining this correction may require the assistance of a healthcare practitioner who can do deeper and more extensive corrections on your system.

Let's test for another possible reversal. Bend forward another time or two to loosen up and get a baseline. Say, "I want to invest at least five hours a week in improving my health." Then bend forward again. As long as you are congruent with that phrase, you will bend forward at least as far as your baseline level.

If you did not bend as far as your baseline when you said this statement, treat this reversal by tapping the reversal point on the edge of your hands together while you say aloud, "I want to invest at least five hours a week into improving my health." After you have done the tapping while verbalizing the statement for about thirty seconds, retest yourself. Say the sentence one more time aloud without tapping, and then do the forward-bending test. If your self-treatment was effective, you should bend at least as far as your baseline, which indicates you are now congruent with this phrase. I suggest you do this tapping at least once a day for the next month or so and monitor yourself to make sure you don't have a recurrence of the reversal.

A reversal is also a strong possibility to consider if you feel stuck along the way or find yourself struggling with following your health plan. Reversals can occur for a number of reasons. One possibility is that you may have additional reversals that are either deeper or are associated with health and success. Reversals can recur on people who have food allergies when they eat foods they are sensitive to. Just know that psychological reversals are common, and it is a good idea to check for them if you find yourself struggling in any particular area.

If you have any reversals or experience a recurrence of them, work with a health professional who can do much more comprehensive corrections. What I have described above is only the tip of the iceberg. The professionals, who work much more deeply at correcting reversals, usually use diagnostic muscle testing to monitor the body's responses and then treat various reflexes to normalize the body's circuitry. They can often find a common denominator that corrects several reversals by improving the function of the body. They are primarily Applied Kinesiologists or practitioners of Neuro-Emotional Technique. They can assist you and greatly increase your chances of continued success. To say it another way, any reversals that are related to health, success, or deserving a good life can sabotage the success of your health plan. Do what you can to not have reversals that could be working against you.

Are you ready to make your health plan a reality? Then let's move ahead and explore "Getting It Right."

7

GETTING IT RIGHT:
EAT, PLAY, AND THINK YOURSELF TO HEALTH

You've committed to investing at least 10 percent of your weekly leisure time into promoting your health. Now let's look at ways to optimize your investment of time so the benefits to you accumulate week after week, year after year, without setbacks that could slow or stop your progress.

Setbacks become costly and frequently cause people to give up on their exercise goals. You may have had similar experiences in which you worked hard at something, saw no results, or perhaps felt worse as a result of your efforts. Naturally, that kind of negative feedback is not going to sustain you, especially when there are so many distractions and pressures in daily life.

Rather than dwelling on what not to do, let's focus on what to do and how you can avoid major pitfalls that cause people to abandon the pursuit of health. Your success may also inspire a couch potato or two to rejoin the ranks of the living and active.

First, let's look at a simple way to pursue your health plan with a high probability of success. Your body's Inner Pharmacy uses the chemical building blocks, the raw materials you provide it, to make necessary chemicals. Your activities, both mental and physical, determine which chemicals your body produces from the available raw materials. It really is that simple, as long as your body is functioning properly, to perform each of these vital functions.

Your Inner Pharmacy produces anti-inflammatory chemicals, just as it produces chemicals that aggravate inflammation. Your body produces chemicals that lower blood pressure, just as it produces ones that raise blood pressure. Your body knows how to control blood-sugar levels so you don't become diabetic, but it has to function properly, have the right raw materials, and not be given an inordinate amount of dietary sugar to control. Your body can break down its own cholesterol and convert it into either high-stress chemicals or stress-reducing chemicals. The body preferentially makes different chemicals, based on what it prioritizes as its needs.

All of this means the choice is yours.

With your health plan, you focus on health and do things that encourage your body to make more good chemicals and fewer bad ones.

Or you could wait. You could ignore your Inner Pharmacy while your bad chemicals exceed your good ones, year after year, and eventually disease develops. Then you can go to your neighborhood pharmacy and buy the good chemicals that your body can't produce. You can also buy other chemicals to counteract the bad ones you are producing in excess. And you can engage in the debate over who is going to pay for your store-bought chemicals, as if it is someone else's responsibility to provide you with the chemicals that you were too lazy or too preoccupied to work on producing yourself.

Besides your improved quality of life, it makes economic sense, both for yourself and as an inhabitant of this planet, to focus on creating your health rather than on treating your disease. You won't see advertisements for your health plan on television, because there aren't a lot of economic interests based on the effective function of your Inner Pharmacy. There is much more interest in selling you the chemicals produced by drug companies.

There are three basic aspects to "getting it right": first, the raw materials you give to your body; second, your mental and physical activities, which determine what your body does with those raw materials; and third, a properly functioning body, which is critical, not just for your day-to-day activities, but to allow you to perform and benefit from health-promoting activities. Let's look at the properly functioning body first.

Maintenance Healthcare

In part 2, we discussed how healthcare can attain and maintain the proper function of the body. To refresh your new perspective and to reinforce your health plan, ask yourself this question:

Do you have regular maintenance done periodically on your car?

Presumably the answer is yes, and you do because you know that your car runs better, is safer, lasts longer, and has less chance of breaking down on you. Right? Now for the next question:

*Do you have regular maintenance done periodically
on your own body?*

If the answer is no, as it probably is, it means that you take better care of your car than your own body. Yet which one of the two could not be replaced if it gave out or totally broke down on you? The point is that most active bodies need periodic maintenance. Just as an example, here is another question:

Have you have ever sprained an ankle?

Furthermore, have you sprained the same ankle more than once? By the way, there are several reasons why people often sprain the same ankle repeatedly. One of them is because the ligaments are injured in the initial sprain. Another is that the muscles which would normally support the ankle are injured as well and often are not able to reset themselves. A third is that the bones in the ankle are frequently misaligned by the sprain. And if uncorrected, the misalignment may remain for many years and deteriorate the function of the ankle so that it no longer absorbs shock properly. This means that the impact of walking or running then sends much more shock into the knee, hip, and low back, causing premature degeneration in those joints. It is not that much different from driving a car with worn-out shock absorbers and then seeing your tires and suspension rapidly wear out.

If there were a way to realign the ankle and to reset the ankle-supporting muscles after an ankle injury, wouldn't it make sense to have that done? There is a way to do precisely that, and it is done routinely on people who see doctors who realign bones and reset muscles, reflexes, and circuits that have been disturbed by injuries or the stresses of daily living. *So many mechanical injuries to the body are fixable.* It just requires knowing that the option exists for maintaining your body and making it a priority to slow the aging process and to extend the life of your parts. Many doctors of different types, especially chiropractors, naturopaths, osteopaths, and acupuncturists, work to restore and to improve the normal function of the body. This is a different paradigm than treating disease. It is wellness-care. It is healthcare in the new landscape of chronic disease.

Sooner or later, people will discover that, as valuable and necessary as they are, drugs and surgery are not the first line of intervention for chronic health problems. Restoring health is the first line of treatment, which means restoring normal function to the body *and* creating a healthy lifestyle to maintain and support that normal function.

As a holistic doctor, I started practice over twenty-five years ago with phenomenal techniques from chiropractic and Applied Kinesiology that correct and restore normal function to the body. Over the years, I have learned how important lifestyle is. Patients with unhealthy lifestyles make it very difficult to maintain normal function in their bodies. Their lifestyles were sometimes beating up and wearing down their bodies faster than I could fix them. On the other hand, patients with healthy lifestyles typically responded better and faster to treatment and maintained the improved function. I learned the important role of the physician as a teacher, and I can tell you that a healthy lifestyle and a properly functioning body go hand in hand. A healthy lifestyle helps to maintain a properly functioning body, and a properly functioning body is necessary to lead and obtain the benefits from a healthy lifestyle.

Since you will be increasing your physical activity, it's essential that you *make exercise your ally*. And that requires the proper function of your body's biomechanics, including shock absorption, muscle function to support and protect your joints, and spinal alignment with freely moving vertebrae so your discs can benefit. You may not know that after the age of around twenty-five, your spinal discs no longer have a blood supply. Their health is maintained by motion that compresses them and eliminates waste products as you move one way and sucks in nutrients from the surrounding tissues as you move another way. It is essential that the vertebrae above and below a disc be in good alignment and moving freely for the disc to receive any benefits from activity. One of the huge benefits from periodic chiropractic spinal adjustments is the improved alignment and motion of the vertebrae, which then helps to keep the discs alive and to slow their degeneration. You don't even have to have back pain as a prerequisite to obtain these benefits.

The best way for you to maintain a properly functioning body is through healthcare. Since most traditional doctors have their hands full with sick people, they have to focus on disease care. You will probably want to work with someone in complementary or alternative care, and I wholeheartedly suggest that you consult with a healthcare doctor, a wellness doctor, who can adjust, treat, and reset areas of your body that are weak links. It will even help you to get out of the grip of saber-toothed tigers and help to change your view of the present moment and what is really important in your life.

Everyone has weak links from their genetic inheritance, from old injuries, and from various stresses and lifestyle imbalances. Strengthen your weak links. Improve the balance in your autonomic nervous system and the function of your digestive system. Maximize your diaphragm muscle function and increase your energy level while getting more oxygen to your brain. Get your body functioning better and have periodic maintenance to keep it functioning better. Make optimal function your goal. Even if you never attain it, you will be heading in the right direction and improving many aspects of your health. And that's a lot better than ignoring the enormous role you can play in improving your quality of life and creating time for your future.

This is true healthcare: caring for your health. It is different from waiting to get sick and then using medical care to treat your sickness.

It is also different from some people's idea of prevention, which only takes the form of "early detection." True prevention is not just having your blood pressure or blood sugar tested periodically to see if you have a problem. True prevention is living a healthy lifestyle that minimizes the chances of developing blood-sugar, cardiovascular, and inflammatory problems. Use all the prevention and early detection that you are able to. Just don't stop there. Don't assume that periodic medical evaluations are themselves going to improve your health. It is very wise for you to have a smoke detector in your house. But having a smoke detector has little to do with you and your family following principles and living in a safe way that minimizes the chance of starting a fire. Take a proactive approach to your health.

Recognize that your "health plan" is different from health insurance. Most traditional health insurance exists to cover medical expenses in the event of injury and disease. Yet referring to it as health insurance gives many people a false sense of security. The misconception that they are "covered," that their health is somehow "ensured," makes it easy to think that nothing else needs to be done. *Understand the difference between treating disease and creating health.*

If you are able to avoid major accidents and life-threatening diseases, you will likely make it to ages sixty-five, seventy-five, eighty-five, or more. But the big question is, *in what condition?* Do you want to arrive at those ages refreshed, healthy, and able to enjoy life? Following your health plan can make all the difference. Make it an *action step* in your health plan to develop a healthcare support system for yourself. You will be increasing the success of everything else that you do in your program. Healthcare that enhances a *properly functioning body* is a critical component of "getting it right."

Healthful Raw Materials

Consuming healthful foods doesn't take a lot more time than consuming unhealthful foods. Healthful eating may require a little more time in shopping and meal preparation and maybe even additional time for you to chew your food properly rather than inhale it. But the time is still not significantly different from the time it takes to

188

buy and prepare unhealthful foods. Realize that healthful eating may be easier than you think. It does not require you to prepare your meals from scratch.

If you made two lists, one of healthful foods and one of unhealthful foods, most items on the lists would be obvious. Healthful foods are whole foods such as fruits, vegetables, meat, fish, and poultry. There may be some differences of opinion on milk and dairy products, red meat, and eggs, but these are healthy in moderation for most people. For a good diet, it may not be necessary to consume them, but they are not inherently harmful to everyone.

Then there are the man-made foods like breads, muffins, cereals, and pastas, and most of us don't even question whether they are good or bad. This last group of highly concentrated, refined carbohydrate foods is usually only scrutinized when someone is on a weight-loss diet and is counting calories and carbohydrates. Since people normally think of a diet as a program to be followed for the purpose of weight reduction, I want to emphasize that a diet in its true sense is simply the collection of raw materials you provide your body to improve your health and to give your Inner Pharmacy good raw materials to work with. Given that you are already on a diet, you may want to modify it to emphasize foods that will improve your health today as well as twenty and thirty years from today.

Many different diets exist, some as a weight-loss plan and some to help a certain condition such as high blood pressure or cholesterol, asthma, diabetes, or cardiovascular disease. There are low and high roughage diets for different intestinal conditions. Bland diets can help to minimize irritation of the stomach and intestines. Diets based on blood types can help to minimize low-grade allergic reactions and guide people to eat good foods that they are unlikely to react to.[1] Body-type diets, based on an individual's glandular makeup, encourage people to eat in a way that improves their health and weight distribution by promoting balance in the endocrine system.[2]

You can easily get lost in the world of diet options and not know where to begin. The ideal approach would take into account any specific condition or health problem, or a strong genetic predisposition for a specific condition, and even the fact that your ideal diet may change over time. I suggest you explore diets and work with a health-care practitioner who can monitor you and guide you to the best diet.

Specific conditions and genetic factors aside, some general dietary guidelines apply to almost everyone. The two most common dietary offenders in Western cultures are excesses of carbohydrates and bad fats. These two alone are responsible for much of the cardiovascular disease, diabetes, and arthritis as well as the rampant obesity that exists today.

Carbohydrates

Carbohydrates or sugars provide important fuel for the body and naturally come in the form of fruits and vegetables grown from the earth. The amount and concentration of carbohydrate vary considerably among different fruits and vegetables. Starches—such as rice, potatoes, and corn—have higher sugar content than complex carbohydrates, such as most green vegetables. And refined carbohydrates—such as most breads, pastas, and packaged wheat products—have a much higher concentration of sugars than any naturally occurring foods.

When you consume more carbohydrates than you burn up for fuel, your body then stores much—at least 40 percent of the excess—as fat. Hence, much weight gain is due to excess carbohydrate consumption, as you probably know. But here's what many people fail to recognize. Excess carbohydrate consumption creates other enormous problems for people, even those who are not overweight. Artificially concentrated carbohydrates create the same hormonal and neuro-chemical changes in your body as when you are being attacked by a saber-toothed tiger. You subject your body to a high-stress event each time you consume a lot of carbohydrates, especially the refined type. The stress and hormonal changes can be taking a huge toll, even if you have no problem with weight gain.

Furthermore, the burst of energy obtained from refined carbo-hydrates is short-lived. It rarely lasts more than a few hours, if that long, and you are left with a craving for more carbohydrates. The average Westerner who consumes 150 pounds of refined sugar each year is caught in this addictive cycle of needing sugar every few hours just to keep going. Remember, healthy aging is an endurance event, and you can't rely on repeated episodes of short bursts of energy to get there. It's not only inefficient, it's damaging in the process. For your physical and mental well-being, minimize your consumption of refined carbohydrates, be moderate with your consumption of starches, and eat more complex carbohydrates like fruits and vegetables.

Carbohydrates are not inherently bad. In their natural state, they provide many nutrients and are a great source of energy. What is bad for health are the processing and concentration of them into manufactured foods, the advertising of these products as healthy, and inordinate consumption.

Fats

A similar misunderstanding exists about dietary fats, which were given a bad reputation in the 1980s and early 1990s, when the trend became high-carbohydrate and low-fat. People got the message that fat was somehow bad for you and had to be avoided. That erroneous concept, accompanied by excess carbohydrate consumption, created much of the chronic illness we see today. Let me say emphatically that fat is not bad for you! While bad fats are bad for you, good fats are very good for you. In fact, the biochemical name for naturally occurring dietary fats is essential fatty acids. They are essential because they are required for vital body functions and cannot be manufactured in the body itself.

The confusion about whether fat is good or bad for you has been complicated by the artificial processing of fats to increase their marketability and shelf life. Fortunately, most of us are now aware of the term trans fats—oils that are artificially hydrogenated—and while we may not understand the chemistry of what it means, we recognize that trans fats can be harmful to the body and are best avoided. I can add that there is simply no way for the Inner Pharmacy to produce good chemicals from trans fats!

Though fats in their natural form are not inherently bad, some can only be tolerated in small amounts while others can be consumed freely and still provide benefits. Since some are clearly better than others, it is accurate to say that all fats are not created equal. More on that later.

191

Further, the ratios of consumption between different dietary fats determines the ratios of pro- and anti-inflammatory chemicals that the Inner Pharmacy can produce, which then results in increased or decreased levels of inflammation. Everyone has the inflammation issue to deal with; where the inflammation occurs depends on genetic factors and localized wear and tear. Knowing and implementing a few basics about different types of fats can help your body control inflammation without the potential side effects and gastrointestinal damage of store-bought anti-inflammatory medications. Done properly, *food can be your best medicine.*

There are three basic categories of fats. Since the technical names are not relevant for a general understanding of the concept, we'll call them fats one, two, and three. Each type that you consume is converted by your Inner Pharmacy into chemicals that affect your body in ways including inflammation, blood clotting, and blood pressure.

Chemicals produced from fats one and three have the qualities of reducing inflammation, lowering blood pressure, and improving circulation, while the chemicals produced from fats two actually increase inflammation, blood pressure, and blood clotting. The amount of each of these chemicals produced by your Inner Pharmacy is a direct result of the amount of fat you consume from each category and the presence of other specific nutrients necessary for some of the chemical conversions—the chemical reactions that convert the food into the chemical which affects the body's physiology.

You can influence the amount of pro- or anti-inflammatory chemicals that your Inner Pharmacy produces through the fats that you consume and by ensuring that you have specific nutrients available to allow for converting those fats into good chemicals. A healthy diet would contain an abundance of fats one and three and a minimum of fats two.

Yet the average Western diet is exactly the opposite! Most of us grow up consuming an abundance of fats two and a minimum of fats one and three. Trans fats, which are widely consumed, are not nutritional fats and don't even fit into any of the categories. Furthermore, the consumption of trans fats wreaks havoc with the Inner Pharmacy and blocks the conversion of fats one and three into good chemicals, thus eliminating their potential good effects. To add insult to injury, a high-carbohydrate intake and the resulting high insulin production also creates a chemical that shifts category one fats into twos and thus increases the production of bad chemicals.

The result, globally, is a huge amount of devastating chronic disease, premature aging, and loss of quality of life. The excess inflammation creates arthritis in one person, cardiovascular disease in another, and a host of conditions whose names end in "itis" running rampant throughout the population.

I haven't revealed yet which fats are within each of the three categories, because I want you to understand the principle without your food preferences or prejudices clouding the issue. I also want you to understand that the challenge is to have a balance of fats in your diet. While it may seem the ideal approach would be to eliminate consumption of fats two and consume lots of fats one and three, it is the ratio of the total of ones and threes versus the twos that is most important. Yes, you want less category-two fats and more ones and threes plus the right conditions for your body to convert ones and threes into good chemicals. Now let's look at what that means.

Category-one fats (omega-6 fats) include most vegetable oils, like olive, safflower, sesame, peanut, almond, corn, and canola. Category-two fats are found in dairy products (milk and butter), meat, and eggs. Category-three fats (omega-3 fats) come from fish and beans. Within each category, some are better for certain situations than others.

A healthful diet, for most people, includes some fat from each category, and with the amounts of ones and threes exceeding the twos. Needless to say, the common imbalance is an excess of twos. Considering that most people are already so out of balance, a good place to start is to make dietary shifts and to add nutritional supplements. Most of us could benefit from more olive oil and fish, especially ocean fish, in our diet. It is also beneficial to supplement with additional oils, like flax seed oil and fish oils, to increase category-three fats. In addition to olive oil, a good supplement for category-one fats is a concentrate of black currant seed oil, because it contains linoleic acid, the active ingredient in that group of fats.

It is all about *balance* and *ratios*. The solution to a healthy ratio is to increase the ones and threes and to decrease the twos. While some purists advise eliminating the twos, my suggestion is to consume them in moderation and with lots of ones and threes to maintain balance. Unless you have some genetic reason or health history to avoid the twos, being healthy doesn't require the elimination of meat, eggs, and dairy products. It simply means not living on them alone.

Balancing your intake of different fats is a good way, over time, to decrease the excess inflammation in your body and to improve your health. Aerobic exercise, done properly and regularly, stimulates the body to burn more fat and increase the conversion of these dietary fats into their respective chemicals which then influence your physiology. It is all very simple, but it has to be done right for it to work.

You might find it interesting to know that one of the ways in which NSAIDs reduce pain and inflammation is by blocking your Inner Pharmacy's ability to convert fats one, two, and three into their respective chemicals that would otherwise affect your physiology. Because they block the conversion of all three categories, and because only the second category of fats causes inflammation, their relief of pain confirms that an excess of category-two fats was a contributing factor to the pain and inflammation. Said another way, if you have an ongoing, continued need for aspirin or other NSAIDs to control your pain and inflammation, there is a high probability you have an ongoing excess of category-two fats and/or a deficiency of category-one and category-three fats.

This is not relevant for the brief and occasional use of NSAIDs to treat injury or an acute problem. But if you take NSAIDs continuously, you would be wise to look at your diet and your fat metabolism. Balancing your fats may not be an overnight correction and may not bring the immediate relief of pain we Americans have been programmed to expect from medications, but it will provide you with huge dividends in quality of life and healthy aging over the long haul.

One more example of the power of dietary fats and their effects on your body can be seen in the class of drugs known as COX 2 inhibitors, one of which is Vioxx, which was taken off the market because of the cardiovascular problems it was causing. This group of drugs works primarily by blocking the conversion of category two fats into their pro-inflammatory chemicals, presumably without affecting category-one and category-three fats. These drugs, an expensive alternative to NSAIDs, are touted as safer because they produce less gastrointestinal side effects and allow you to continue consuming an excess of bad fats or maintaining a deficiency of good fats without experiencing the pain and inflammation normally caused by this imbalance.

While there is a need for safer and more effective medications that produce fewer side effects, there is an even greater need to look at the normal physiology of the body and to use the Inner Pharmacy as the first line of treatment, especially for chronic problems. When this is done, the external pharmacy of manufactured medications can be used, secondarily and as necessary, to augment whatever it is that the body is unable to do on its own. Give your Inner Pharmacy the opportunity to create as many good chemicals as possible. You can safely do that through your own lifestyle. It's called "getting it right."

Several methods, including blood and saliva tests, diet analysis, and Applied Kinesiology, evaluate for specific imbalances of essential fats. These tests are performed by many holistic-thinking and health-promoting doctors, who can give you the most efficient way to optimize your health. The general rule for everyone is this: Eat more good fats and less bad fats, and engage in activities that stimulate your body to convert that good fat into good chemicals.

Proteins

Besides carbohydrates and fats, the other food group that provides critical raw materials for your Inner Pharmacy is proteins. While a general formula exists, the optimal amount of protein intake varies considerably according to body type, amount of physical activity, and the efficiency of one's digestive system, to name just a few factors.

Having said that, protein foods provide essential nutrients and raw materials for the Inner Pharmacy and maintain the normal pH or acid-base balance of the body. Foods with the highest concentration of protein are meat, poultry, fish, eggs, dairy products, beans, and nuts.

It is common for people to exhibit deficiencies in protein, and a close look at their blood tests can confirm it. They often experience painful joints, since proteins normally maintain the smoothness of joint surfaces. Sometimes they are deficient in specific amino acids, the building blocks of proteins, which the body uses to make neurotransmitter chemicals. Since protein is a building block the body uses for many different functions, an active person with a high-stress lifestyle will use up more of certain amino acids than a calm, sedentary person would. The saber-toothed tiger stimulates production of adrenaline and other neurotransmitters, the production of which requires amino acids and vitamins. Unless they take in more of the necessary raw materials, people under chronic high stress use up more amino acids and vitamins and can deplete their supplies.

Since normal digestion is critical for making proteins available for the Inner Pharmacy, another factor that can lead to a protein deficiency is poor stomach function. People with stomach problems or those chronically taking gastric acid–suppressive drugs are more prone to develop protein deficiencies as the years go by. It is common for heartburn and gastric reflux after a meal to be caused, not by excess stomach acid, as often assumed, but by the acid getting up into the esophagus where it does not belong. People are now recognizing that stomach acid has several vital functions, one of which is as a first line of defense by killing bacteria that enter the body and make it to the stomach. Suppressing stomach acid compromises this protective function.

Respect and maintain your good digestive function. If you have symptoms of stomach acid getting up into your esophagus, do something about it. Don't ignore it. But don't just take a medication to suppress your stomach-acid production. Work with a doctor who can improve the function of your diaphragm muscle and esophageal sphincter to help keep the acid down in the stomach where it belongs.

As for digestion of protein, the general rule is to eat moderate amounts each day and digest it well. Do this by relaxing when you eat and not mixing proteins with high-carbohydrate foods like starches and sugars. Even though a meat-and-potatoes meal is a staple in many cultures, you digest proteins better if you have them

196

along with complex carbohydrates like vegetables. It is better to have meat or fish with vegetables rather than with rice, pasta, or potatoes. And as for relaxing, your body can't digest much of anything, especially protein, while you are racing to escape a saber-toothed tiger. The fight-or-flight response turns off normal digestion and stifles your appetite.

For maintenance, I recommend moderate amounts of protein daily. Even for a patient who is protein-deficient, I don't suggest high-protein diets except when used temporarily for weight loss or building muscle. Most high-protein diets include large amounts of category-two fats—those from animal proteins. Unless you are also consuming lots of category-one and category-three fats and getting significant amounts of protein from ocean fish, a high-protein diet over the years can lead to increased inflammation from the excess of category-two fats. High-protein diets also make the kidneys work much harder. If a high-protein diet is consumed temporarily to lose weight, the net health improvements from the weight loss probably exceed the drawbacks. But for healthy aging, energy, and endurance, moderate protein balanced with complex carbohydrates and good fats provides the best array and combination of raw materials for your Inner Pharmacy.

Water and liquids

Many of us don't drink enough water. *A water deficiency may be the biggest nutritional deficiency in the Western world.* It is important for adults to consume at least six to eight eight-ounce glasses of water every day, preferably between meals and preferably not at night before going to bed. Water consumed with a meal can dilute the digestive juices and compromise your ability to properly digest the meal. So, water is not only important, but the timing of when it is drunk is important as well.

Regardless of how much juice, tea, coffee, or other liquid you consume, your body needs water. These other beverages can actually increase your water needs. Water consumption is extremely important for children, and the sooner they learn this lesson the better. If they are conditioned to quench their thirst with juice, soda, or other sweetened drinks, they will choose the artificial sweetness over the plain water. This perpetuates their water deficiency and craving for sweets.

The good news for children or adults whose tastes have been conditioned by frequent consumption of refined sugar and sweetened foods and drinks is that *tastes change.* That's how we get conditioned to want the inordinately sweet taste of highly concentrated sugars and artificial sweeteners in the first place. You didn't come into this world with a natural taste for the extraordinary sweetness found in many manufactured foods and beverages. You acquire that taste from repeated exposure and then came to expect it. Your tastes changed.

It is also easy to change your tastes back. I have worked with hundreds of patients who described themselves as sugar addicts but who nevertheless gave up concentrated sugars and artificial sweeteners. After two to three weeks on a healthy diet, I encourage them to taste a sweet food or drink they had previously enjoyed. Almost universally, after weeks away from sugar, they experience their former favorites as unpleasant and often disgustingly sweet.

In another example, you could taste a piece of fresh watermelon and experience it as pleasantly sweet. But if you consumed a bowl of ice cream or a soft drink first and then tasted the watermelon, you would probably not even recognize its natural sweetness. Tastes are relative, and tastes change, which means you can break an addiction to sugar.

You don't have to be perfect with your diet and lifestyle changes as long as you are moving in the right direction. But if you are frequently (daily) consuming refined carbohydrates, concentrated sugars, or artificially sweetened foods and beverages, the best approach may be to totally eliminate these foods for at least two weeks. Perfect behavior, in this case, may be the easiest and most effective way to tackle the problem. Being strict with your diet for two weeks can break the addiction to the sweetness, allow your tastes to normalize, and give your body a break from having to process all those sugars and artificial chemicals. You will probably find that your sugar craving passes after a few days, and you may find that after two weeks, you are feeling better than you have for a long time. If you feel overwhelmed about what you *cannot* eat, just shift your attention to all the healthful foods you *can* eat. The basic rule is "Eat foods that God made."

Some physical conditions, such as hypoglycemia, may require the assistance of a health-oriented physician to supervise your diet change. Depending on the extent of your cravings for sugar, treatment to normalize your neuroendocrine system can support and ease this transition to a healthy diet. Specific nutritional supplements can also help your Inner Pharmacy normalize your physiology and reduce your sugar cravings. Getting the body to control its own sugar-regulating mechanisms may be easy for some people. But for those who have consumed excess sugar for a long time and for those who have lived high-adrenaline lifestyles for years, getting out of that destructive cycle may be a challenge which requires your total commitment, persistence, and the assistance of healthcare professionals.

Food supplements

No matter how good your diet, it is a wise practice to supplement it with vitamins and other nutrients. How much your diet should be supplemented depends on the quality of your diet and how long you've eaten well (and how long you've eaten poorly), combined with your genetics, lifestyle, current health, and health goals.

Your biochemical individuality determines the ideal set of raw materials your Inner Pharmacy needs to meet the challenges of your daily life while building and not depleting your reserves. Furthermore, the optimum ratios of certain nutrients can preferentially favor the Inner Pharmacy's production of good chemicals over bad ones. Rarely can a diet alone meet these criteria, unless you are in very good health to begin with and are meticulous about food choices, preparation, food combining, and the function of your digestive system.

A nutritious diet would be a lot easier if our agricultural topsoils had not been depleted of minerals and laden with toxic chemicals from decades of chemical-based agricultural practices. The loss of vitality and fertility of our soils is taking a huge toll on human health, and it necessitates additional supplementation of our diets.

At a time when high-stress lifestyles increase people's nutrient requirements, even a good diet of whole foods now contains fewer nutrients to meet those needs.

Also, many manufactured and sugared foods use more of your body's nutrients to process them than they supply. These are "negative foods." Their consumption depletes the body rather than nurtures it as foods should do. Their frequent consumption can easily create nutritional deficiencies.

Specific symptoms can result from a deficiency of one or more nutrients. Accurately identifying the deficiency and providing the nutrients to correct it is a fairly simple and common scenario. This is one use of nutritional supplementation in which there is a specific remedy for a specific problem. But that is not the only reason for taking nutritional supplements.

Because of the interconnectedness of the body's systems, a wide array of nutrients is needed for the body to function normally. A symptom is the result of some underlying dysfunction. Rather than just addressing symptoms, your goal is to promote normal function—to create your good health. The presence of many nutrients enables your body to function normally, whereas the absence or deficiency of one specific nutrient—such as a vitamin, amino acid, trace mineral, or essential fatty acid—can hinder your Inner Pharmacy from completing a chemical reaction. It may be able to adapt to the absence of the needed nutrient and complete the process by an alternative or auxiliary pathway, which may be inefficient and deplete other nutrients in the process. This downward spiral of adaptations accelerates the aging process and predisposes you to further dysfunction and the eventual development of disease.

Having a wide array of raw materials available to your Inner Pharmacy is not the same as having large or unnecessary amounts of any given raw material. The promotion and maintenance of health rarely requires high doses of any nutrient. Actually, the intake of megadoses of vitamins and nutrients is a challenge to regulate, because the high dose of one nutrient may stimulate a certain chemical pathway that then requires higher doses of other nutrients. If the other nutrients are unavailable, again inefficient auxiliary pathways may be the only option and may depend on yet other nutrients that could be unavailable.

There is a big difference between taking megadoses of a few nutrients—an approach I rarely recommend—and the common (and safe) supplementation of low dosages of a variety of high-quality, biologically active nutrients. Most of us will benefit from the latter, which provides many nutrients that are both missing from foods and are increasingly needed due to demanding lifestyles, and which does not overload the body with any one nutrient.

High doses of vitamin E (above 400 IUs a day) may often have many effects opposite to the same vitamin in lower doses. The amount you take determines its effects. For example, while lower doses of vitamin E will often help decrease blood pressure, amounts higher than 400 units a day can raise blood pressure. Lower doses help to decrease inflammation, while higher doses actually block the Inner Pharmacy's production of anti-inflammatory chemicals and lead to further inflammation. Throughout my career, I have reduced the vitamin E intake of many patients who were influenced by the typical "more-is-better" mentality.

Since certain health problems can be aggravated by high doses of vitamin E, some people worry that vitamin E is harmful, which is not true. This misunderstanding then creates a phobia of taking vitamins. One study showed that increased intake of vitamin E did not reduce the incidence of cardiovascular disease or cancer in patients at least fifty-five years old with vascular disease or diabetes, and this was interpreted as meaning that vitamin E is useless.[3] Yet that study did not answer whether a *deficiency* of vitamin E could predispose a healthy person to cardiovascular disease or cancer. Until that question is answered, it is prudent to consume adequate amounts of vitamin E.

A basic array of low-dosage nutrients is both safe and helpful for most people. This recommendation is made, not on individual needs, but on the likelihood that our lifestyles demand these nutrients and that our diets are not sufficiently supplying them. This is a starting place, a set of common denominators that apply to a high percentage of people of all ages.

For the general population, the things I most recommend to supplement a good diet are (1) a multiple vitamin, (2) a B complex, (3) a mineral supplement, and (4) an essential fatty acid supplement, probably fish oils or a complex of the good oils that we discussed earlier.

Start here, but don't stop here. This is just a basic way to supplement a good diet, to provide your Inner Pharmacy with necessary ingredients, and to prevent deficiencies that can cause adaptations now and health problems later on. If, however, you are already out of balance and deficient in some nutrients, it would be best to identify those deficiencies and specifically address them. You can have blood, urine, and saliva tests evaluated by a health professional, who can give specific recommendations to improve your physiology. There is a difference between the conventional review of blood tests from the point of view of ruling out disease and a health-oriented review, which looks toward optimizing body function. I do both and can tell you that a health-oriented review uses much stricter criteria in the evaluation of lab tests.

For complicated health problems, I individually evaluate and test each patient, review thorough lab tests, treat the person to improve the function of the body, and then recommend supplements based on that person's biological individuality. Periodic reevaluations allow me to monitor the patient's progress and make further recommendations. It is an ongoing process of identifying weak links and working to strengthen them. If the treatment, diet, supplements, and lifestyle changes all are working, the lab tests will show the improvements. If the tests are not improving significantly, the strategy is modified.

The better your diet and body function is, the less supplementation you need. It is quite common for people with functional disorders to be deficient in one or more basic nutrients, like zinc, magnesium, thiamine, riboflavin, vitamin D, folic acid, potassium, calcium, and others. Find a healthcare doctor who provides individualized evaluation and can give you a health assessment.

Food sensitivities

Another topic in the discussion of raw materials is food sensitivities, like those seen with John in chapter 4. Because these reactions in the body are not necessarily classic allergic reactions, it is more accurate to refer to them as *sensitivities*. There are several types of "allergic reactions" that can occur in the body. Since some are delayed reactions that are not usually life-threatening, they are often overlooked and can be difficult to identify. They may occur a day or two after a food is eaten, and sometimes they occur only after a food has been eaten repeatedly. Yet they are frequently responsible for causing chronic health problems. Because they trigger reactions that attack different parts of the body, depending on an individual's genes, they are common contributing factors in joint pain, headaches, skin problems, and back pain as well as digestive problems and typical allergies.

If you have some chronic or ongoing pain or another health problem, consider the possibility that something you frequently eat or drink might be triggering a reaction that is creating or perpetuating the problem. Consider also the possibility that if your body is reacting to something you are putting into it and is triggering inflammation in your joints, for example, it may also be triggering inflammation in your blood vessels, your cardiovascular system. Months and years of these reactions create a lot of chronic pain and inflammation, which vastly deteriorates the body and leads many to the long-term use of anti-inflammatory medication.

In the case of food sensitivities, the Inner Pharmacy reacts not as if a normal food has been consumed that can provide useful raw materials but as if that food or drink were some harmful, foreign substance that should not and cannot be properly digested and utilized. The ensuing reactions create bad chemicals that then cause the body to attack itself, which results in the inflammation. The solution is to eliminate the triggers for inflammation and to help the Inner Pharmacy control whatever inflammation does develop through normal wear and tear.

How can you know if any foods are adversely affecting you? Classic allergy testing does not always evaluate for delayed reactions in the body. But lab tests that evaluate either blood, saliva, or both can give an accurate assessment of whether food sensitivities may be a source of your chronic problems. Your healthcare professional can use these tests and others to evaluate whether food sensitivities may be a source of your chronic problems. Since some of these reactions to specific foods are moderated by one's blood type, Dr. Peter J. D'Adamo's blood-type diets in his *Eat Right for Your Type* (New York: G. P. Putnam's Sons, 1996) are helpful for many people.

Food sensitivities often involve a food you eat frequently and/or a food that you crave. If you have a chronic problem, look to your diet for something that might be triggering your problem. By eliminating a food for several weeks, you can see if there is a difference.

Your Five Hours to Good Health

You have already committed to investing 10 percent of your weekly leisure time, or at least five hours a week, into stress-reducing and health-promoting activities. Let's consider ways you can optimize that five hours to create as much balance in your life as possible and to aid your Inner Pharmacy in its vital work.

You now have five hours a week to use in creative, productive ways to improve your health and quality of life! It a significant step to make this commitment, and you may be wondering what you have gotten yourself into. Simple: You will be investing your five hours a week in specific physical and mental activities of your own choosing, meaning that it can be *fun*. It is your health plan, and the only challenge you may have is to maintain your commitment. Just remember to pay yourself first. Schedule these five hours into your weekly calendar. When time conflicts arise, work around your already scheduled appointment with yourself, because you have made it a priority.

It is important to invest at least four of the five hours into physical activity. Because of its enormous mental and physical benefits, spend at least three hours in aerobic activity and one hour in some form of muscle-strength training. Reserve your fifth hour for an activity that reduces your stress and mentally refreshes you. This mental-health hour can inspire you and change your relationship to the saber-toothed tigers that chase you around in daily life.

Aerobic activity

Since it is the largest unit of time investment, let's first look at aerobic activity. Would you like to burn up some body fat and maybe even reduce your cholesterol and blood fats? Would you like to have more energy and increase your Inner Pharmacy's production of anti-inflammatory chemicals? Aerobic activity is fat-burning activity, and you are going to train your body to burn fat.

The degree to which an activity is aerobic depends on your heart rate, or how fast your heart beats during that activity. If your heart rate is either too fast or too slow, the activity becomes less aerobic and more anaerobic, or sugar-burning. There are three components to your aerobic workout: the warm-up, the aerobic range, and the cool-down. Let's first establish the heart rate that will give you the greatest aerobic benefits.

For calculating your ideal aerobic range, use Dr. Maffetone's "180 formula" mentioned in chapter 4. Begin by subtracting your age from 180. Modify this number as follows:

1. Subtract ten, if you have or are recovering from a major illness or are taking any regular medication.

2. Subtract five, if (a) you have not exercised before, (b) you have been exercising but have been injured or are not making progress, or (c) you have allergies or frequently get sick with colds or flu.

3. Subtract zero, if you have been exercising at least four times a week for up to two years without injury and do not get colds or flu more than twice a year.

4. Add five, if you have been exercising for more than two years without injury.

You now have a number that becomes the highest number in a range of ten. This range is your ideal aerobic heart rate, or the rate that optimizes your aerobic function. For example, if you are 40 years old, subtract 40 from 180, which gives you 140. And if you have not exercised in years, then subtract five, which gives you 135 as the highest number in your range of ten, that is, 125 to 135. You should exercise to get your heart beating in the range of 125 to 135 beats per minute, which will get your body to burn more fat and convert it into energy and good chemicals. If you do this for thirty minutes a day, your body also burns more fat in the day's other

23½ hours, even while you sleep, as a result of what you did for that one-half hour.

It takes about twelve to fifteen minutes of activity in your aerobic range to make changes in your liver that increase fat burning. This means you can efficiently exercise in as little as thirty minutes a day, including a five- to seven-minute warm-up, a minimum of fifteen minutes in your range, and a five- to seven-minute cool-down. Both the warm-up and cool-down phases are times of transition during which your heart rate is gradually changing from its resting rate, averaging around seventy-two beats a minute, to your aerobic rate, and back again. The warm-up and cool-down phases are critical, both for your safety and so that you obtain the benefits from your activity.

Misconceptions about warming-up and cooling-down are responsible for many exercise-induced injuries. The average person thinks a warm-up entails stretching muscles or doing some form of loosening up. Warming-up really pertains to changes in your blood circulation when you go from a resting heart rate to an exercising heart rate. At your resting heart rate, a certain percentage of your blood is being sent to your muscles and another percentage is being sent to your internal organs, including your heart and brain. At your aerobic exercise rate, a greater percentage of blood is being sent to your muscles. This means that less blood is being sent to your internal organs while you maintain the higher heart rate. So the transition from a resting heart rate to an exercise heart rate is really one of diverting some of the blood supply from your internal organs to your muscles. When a proper warm-up is ignored and the transition to an aerobic heart rate is too rapid, two types of serious injuries can occur. First, muscles are much more prone to sprain or strain if the body has not yet increased the blood circulation to them. Second, the abrupt diversion of blood away from your heart, brain, and other internal organs is potentially dangerous. We have all heard stories of someone who started off on a run and suffered a heart attack. Often accompanying those unfortunate events is a failure to warm up properly.

Train your body to safely and efficiently transition into these circulatory changes, both in the warm-up and cool-down phases. A gradual cool-down of at least five to seven minutes means a smooth diversion of the extra blood supply from muscles back to your internal organs. This allows the muscles to more efficiently eliminate waste products that built up during exercise and greatly reduces the stiff, achy sensations and the increased risk of injury to muscles that were not allowed to properly cool down. If you allocate forty-five minutes or more to your aerobic exercise sessions with a gradual twelve- to fifteen-minute warm-up and cool-down on each side of fifteen minutes in your aerobic range, the benefits increase. The transition times will contribute greatly to the development and increased efficiency of your aerobic (fat-burning) system. But you don't have to limit the time in your aerobic range to fifteen minutes. Thirty or more minutes will increase your fat burning, as long as you maintain your aerobic heart rate.

If you have been accustomed to exercising at a higher heart rate or without a warm-up, you may think you aren't even exercising at this heart rate and may wonder how you could possibly be accomplishing anything. When you exercised previously, the higher heart rate gave you the adrenaline rush, because it was anaerobic, or sugar-burning, and it stimulated your body to do the same things it does when attacked by a saber-toothed tiger. You may have gotten your exercise high, burned some calories, and toned some muscles, but at what expense to your body? With the right genetics and strong adrenal glands, you may be able to continue this for years without injury. Yet it is only efficient for short bursts of activity, and it actually inhibits your body's fat-burning and endurance capabilities. At some point, exercising without warm-ups and cool-downs will produce more fatigue, episodes of low blood-sugar, and increased cortisol, which often creates anxiety and sleep problems. On top of that, your chances of musculoskeletal pain and injury are greater. Sugar-burning exercise increases your need for additional nutrients and ultimately becomes one more high-stress event in the course of your day.

Contrast this with the aerobic exercise that refreshes you and produces more energy and anti-inflammatory chemicals by training your body to burn fat. Your exercise is stress-reducing, offsetting the day's stresses rather than adding to them. You may not experience an adrenaline rush while exercising with a proper warm-up and cool-down, and frankly, you shouldn't. If that sounds like a deterrent, reflect on why you exercise in the first place and what you hope to attain from it. Health and fitness are not the same. You can be very fit and unhealthy at the same time. But if you follow the exercise plan described in this chapter, you can improve your fitness and health at the same time. It just requires following certain principles and exercising with continuity to obtain the health dividends.

Remember, you will be doing aerobic exercise for at least three hours every week. Choose an activity that enables you to gradually increase your heart rate and maintain it in your range. Common activities that fit these criteria are walking, running, cycling, swimming, skating/blading, rowing, and aerobics classes (although they tend toward higher heart rates that are often anaerobic).

Two guidelines that help make exercise a painless endeavor are, first, choose something you enjoy, and second, whatever that is, feel positive about doing it. The more you can make it enjoyable and fun, the more you will look forward to it and experience it as a high point in your day, and the more physical and mental benefits you will receive.

Alternating between different activities is a good idea, like walking/ running for three thirty-minute sessions and cycling for three. You could do six thirty-minute sessions or four forty-five-minute sessions a week and still total your three hours of aerobic activity. Choose any combination of times and activities, as long as you have a minimum fifteen minutes in your range and the proper warm-up and cool-down each time. If you can do more than three hours a week, it's even better. Just be sure to schedule your three hours minimum each week into your daily planner, and maintain your commitment.

I recommend using a heart-rate monitoring device. The easiest kind consists of a wristwatch that receives a signal from a strap worn around the chest. The signal corresponds to the heart rate. These devices can be purchased at most sporting-goods stores or through my website, *www.start2health.com*. Get a simple, inexpensive monitor, although if you plan on swimming, you'll need a waterproof one. More complicated monitors with various functions are great to work up to or for dedicated athletes in training. But I have seen people give up on heart-rate monitoring because they got frustrated with high-end monitors that were not user-friendly for beginners. Good and simple ones can be purchased for under $100 and are an investment that can last many years.

Muscle strengthening and flexibility

The other hour of physical activity can be devoted to strengthening muscles and increasing your flexibility. Activities aimed at strengthening muscles also help to maintain bone strength and resiliency and can have a positive effect on stimulating your metabolism. More than an hour a week in these activities results in more gains. This category of activity can be addressed in many ways, including traditional weight training, active yoga sessions, and even Pilates classes. The hour a week minimum could be met through one hour-long session, two half-hour sessions, or even ten minutes a day, six days a week.

If you aren't sure what you want to do, explore your options. Contact a local health club or a personal trainer to pursue the weight-training possibility. Most clubs have free passes and introductory packages to allow people to get acquainted with their facilities. Attend an introductory yoga class. While you can learn about yoga from a book, attending a class is safer and more efficient, and it will provide you with an experience that may be much different from what you expected. The number of yoga enthusiasts is growing by the thousands every year as people discover its physical stimulation and calming, centering effects. It could easily become one of the high points of your week. Pilates sessions are particularly good if you want to improve your core muscle strength, carriage, and posture, or if you have been physically injured and want to rehabilitate yourself. Explore the options, and do something on a regular basis that adds up to at least one hour a week. Once you decide on what you will do for this category, put it on your weekly calendar.

The mental-health hour

The mental category is flexible; tailor it to your personality and preferences. What is relaxing and stress-reducing for one person may be torture for someone else. The goal is simply to give yourself one hour totally free from any saber-toothed tigers or even thoughts of them. This hour is for you to just *be*, to live time in the present, to immerse yourself in something inspirational that you enjoy.

The effect of not feeling out of control, rushed, or frantic, even for an hour, can shift your Inner Pharmacy to change your brain chemistry. You are, in effect, changing your relationship to the tigers.

Look at the word *recreation*, which really means *re-creation*. The more destructive your lifestyle is to your health and well-being, the more recreation you need to keep from falling apart. Fortunately, most of us find diversions that provide opportunities to refresh ourselves and to adjust our mind-set. True recreation, however, is not just diversion. It is restorative to health and renews the human spirit. I know people who insist that shopping or watching a football game does this for them, and perhaps it does. Don't worry; I'm not recommending that you go shopping or watch football for an hour a week.

Instead, explore activities that are relaxing, that are inspirational, and that involve some dynamic "life energy." This may sound a bit paradoxical, but let me give some examples. Massage, meditation, and relaxation techniques are perfect for this category. Play, which most adults have forgotten how to do, also fits, as long as it is play without competition. It's not that competition isn't good, but most adults are unable to compete at anything without activating their adrenal stress mechanisms. The purpose of this category is to inactivate those stress mechanisms. Immersing yourself in nature with a hike or a walk in a park can be quite relaxing and inspirational for many, while others might feel bored and restless. There are tremendous benefits from resonating with natural frequencies, which is part of what happens to us in natural environments. Cultural experiences like live music, theater, and art are good fits for many people. Everyone connects with nature and life energy in some way. Choose activities that develop this connection.

A good film or even a good book would be a stretch for this category, as is listening to prerecorded music. These may be great activities, but they don't quite take you enough out of the norm of everyday activities unless they are truly exceptional experiences. If you really feel that one of these constitutes the absolutely most relaxing and stress-reducing way you could use that hour, go ahead and include it.

Some activities fit in more than one health-promoting category. Most forms of yoga could potentially fit all the categories, as it contains invigorating, toning, and aerobic components as well as calming ones providing specific mental stress reduction, and it improves muscle strength and flexibility as well. You might prefer to invest your full five hours a week in the practice of yoga. Yet it would be even better to have at least one or two of those hours go to different activities for diversity and to keep it dynamic and interesting.

Make a list of some of your favorite recreational activities—ones that leave you relaxed, refreshed, and inspired. Schedule at least an hour a week for one of them. Alternate them if you like, but put one or more of them into your weekly planner and keep your appointment with yourself.

Health-Planning Summary

1. You are investing time to create time. Specifically, invest at least 10 percent of your leisure time each week into health-promoting activities. That time investment will improve your health, which is how you create a future and the quality time to enjoy it. Healthy living also brings immediate benefits, such as improved productivity and an enhanced quality of life.

2. You now have a health plan, including a list of your health assets and liabilities and your health-related goals for ages sixty-five, seventy-five, and eighty-five.

3. You are congruent with wanting to be healthy and wanting to invest at least five hours a week into improving your health. If you find yourself not following through on your commitment or sabotaging the success of your health plan, it is likely that you have become psychologically reversed. Self-test using the forward-bending test, or just tap on the hand points while saying the positive statements. If reversals recur, it is best to work with a health professional who can reset your circuitry in a deeper way. Do whatever it takes to maintain your focus and your weekly investments in health.

211

4. Work with a health doctor who can help you identify and strengthen any weak links in your body. Establish a maintenance schedule that continues to optimize your function. Create and maintain wellness for yourself. Remember, it's not "You are what you eat." It's "You are what you absorb," and that totally depends on how well your body is functioning.

5. Consume healthy nutrients through both your diet and nutritional supplements. Give your Inner Pharmacy the raw materials it needs to produce good chemicals. If you have ongoing, chronic problems, consider and investigate the possibility that something you regularly consume may be triggering a reaction in your body and creating your problems.

6. Drink lots of water, which is best done between meals.

7. Schedule at least five hours each week in your weekly planner, and use those five hours to improve your health. It is best to establish a consistent routine for at least three or four of the hours. If that is impossible, schedule your five hours differently each week depending on your other commitments. Each of these hours is, at the very least, an appointment with yourself. If you absolutely need to reschedule, do so. But reschedule for that week and keep your appointments. It is efficient to schedule a month at a time or at least to establish a specific time each week to schedule the following week's appointments. Sundays or evenings are often a good time for this.

8. These five hours can highly influence your Inner Pharmacy to produce good chemicals from the raw materials you give it. At least three of the hours should go into aerobic activity, and you will want to obtain a heart-rate monitor. Make it a gift to yourself or just think of it as a wise investment, which is exactly what it is. One of the hours goes into muscle-strength training. The fifth hour is recreational and is devoted to activities that mentally refresh, renew, and inspire you.

So, there you have it—a simple plan to follow. Your plan can extend your life and the life of your parts. Your new lifestyle will not eliminate but will postpone and delay much of the age-related decline in health that can seriously deteriorate quality of life. In doing so, you actually create quality time—in the only way possible. Invest your time wisely.

Graduation Celebration

Honor your accomplishments after the first month of living your health plan. Have a little graduation celebration! Though you may still be exploring different health-promoting activities, healthcare professionals, and improvements to your diet, the completion of your first month is monumental. You will have completed the most challenging part of health planning, which is maintaining your commitment to yourself. You will already be experiencing the benefits of your new program, and that is just the beginning! You will have established the routine of a healthy lifestyle, will be using healthcare in a whole new way, and will be regularly investing at least 10 percent of your leisure time into your health fund, which will continue to grow, to mature, and to be there for you, providing time and quality of life when you are ready to make some withdrawals.

Your real graduation, however, will take place on your sixty-fifth, seventy-fifth, and eighty-fifth birthdays when your health fund matures and, barring unforeseen circumstances, you achieve your goals and truly experience the value of quality time and healthy living. Whatever your condition when you arrive at those landmark birthdays, it will be much greater than it would have been had you not created and followed a health plan that nurtures your Inner Pharmacy.

EPILOGUE

Your health plan and your new lifestyle are much more significant than you may realize. What you are now doing is monumental: You are not only improving your own health and quality of life, you are supporting a long-overdue shift in how we approach health and disease, a shift which is very near its tipping point. Health and maintaining a youthful vitality throughout life can be quite contagious. You are adding to the critical mass that will have infinite positive effects on the health of our nation and even the world.

As stated in chapter 1, in the spring of 2004, the World Health Organization met in Geneva and acknowledged two earthshaking global shifts: one, the world now has more overweight people than malnourished people; and two, infectious diseases are no longer responsible for most of the world's deaths.[1] With the great strides made in the control of infectious diseases, this global shift raises the question, "Where do we go from here?" The pharmaceutical and technological advancements that got us this far are not the sole solution to our next set of challenges. Our next set of challenges has more to do with chronic disease than acute disease. It has as much to do with problems from excesses of the wrong foods as it does with deficiencies of the right foods.

It is time for a course correction. Creating health has to take precedence over treating disease. And it is that simple. We don't have to abandon everything we know about treating disease; we can honor and utilize those mighty developments. We must simply add to them everything we know about creating health. We must shift our attention to the creation of health first. Then, when it is necessary, we can treat disease. Yet since there is no centralized, organized group that makes money from a mass of people becoming healthy, you may not be hearing this message everyday.

Since you have read and hopefully followed my recommendations on health planning and healthy living and will continue following your plan, I want you to understand what it really means. I teach classes, tutor other doctors, and encourage health planning, and I wrote this book because it is my responsibility as a physician to educate, to share the truth, and to give people options for pursuing the truth. As a holistic doctor, my perspective has been slanted toward correcting the body so it can function normally and heal itself as well as toward educating and guiding patients to a healthy lifestyle so they are not excessively deteriorating the normal function of the body. Getting people healthy is one thing. Keeping them healthy is another, and this is frequently much more difficult than it should be. The biggest reasons for the difficulty can often be traced to deeply ingrained cultural attitudes about health and disease.

Here is a prime example of a common attitude toward aging. Typically, when someone experiences a painful joint, the first response might be, "Well, I guess I'm getting older." If the joint pain continues and expands to other joints, the common response is, "I must have arthritis; therefore, I need a medication." The questions then become, "Which medication should I take?" and "Who is going to pay for it?" This is the typical old "treat the disease" approach that many of us attempt to apply to chronic disease because it worked so well for acute and infectious diseases.

We are all subject to those attitudes. Yet in creating and implementing your health plan, not only do you disconnect yourself from some of the old attitudes about disease, but you help to reinforce new attitudes about health. Let's take that same joint pain and ask a different set of questions from a perspective of health. The first questions to ask are, "Is something malfunctioning in my body? If so, what is it and what can be done to correct it?" The next questions are, "What is triggering my problem? Is it something I am doing or possibly something I am not doing?" Another question is, "Who can help me to answer these questions, to improve the function of my body, and to guide me to do whatever it takes to correct the problem?"

Can you see the difference? Still, every day, children and adults who watch television receive thousands of messages programming them to think a certain way about their need for one medication after another. In the future, each time you are exposed to advertising for medications, simply change your response. Instead of immediately thinking, "Do I need that medication?" ask yourself if there is a way you may be able to get your Inner Pharmacy to produce more of the good chemicals and less of the bad chemicals in order to help your body regulate the symptoms in question.

If you are thinking of beginning to take an optional medication for a long time, perhaps for life, for a chronic problem, you may want to do your own cost/benefit analysis. Be sure to include the high cost of potentially harmful side effects. People are deeply indoctrinated to believe that it is OK to compromise their present and future health from side effects as long as they get relief from their current symptoms now. Looking at your options is much bigger than just asking for another, safer medication to get rid of your symptoms; it's about being healthy. And the benefits of being healthy take on a life of their own and carry a lot of weight when properly factored into any cost/benefit discussion.

When the focus is on health first, a shift occurs from "What medication should I take" to "What can I do?" Instead of running from tigers, your focus is on moving toward health. Instead of survival mode, it's planning for and creating the future you want.

There is a need for massive change in our approach to health and disease, and a course correction is imminent. Whether you realize it or not, the massive "healthcare" industry is ultimately consumer-driven. Much of the trillions of dollars spent on healthcare is highly influenced by deeply held cultural attitudes and beliefs. As people shift more attention to health, so does the economy. Your choices drive the markets. The enormous growth in the use of complementary and alternative medicine occurred because millions of us chose to use these services. And we did so not only for the results but because alternative medicine is more congruent with our philosophy of health and wholeness.[2]

When health and quality time become your priorities, you'll see many issues from a different perspective. From the real costs of poisoning our environment to the depletion of nutrients in our foods through chemical agricultural practices, from funding for the arts that help us to be more balanced and well-rounded people to funding for physical education and athletic programs that teach youth the importance of physical activity—all become obvious and urgent priorities when the health of a nation is our goal.

As you continue to follow your health plan and encourage others to make and follow their own, your life and their lives will change for the better. Let others know that it is never too late to start. Maintain and renew your intention to be healthy, and continue to create a lifestyle and a healthcare support system that nurtures you and your loved ones. Everyone will do this a little differently but with the same common denominators. Your biochemical individuality means that you have to explore options to discover what works for you. Some healthcare professionals place a great emphasis on the matching process and can help you in directing your own healthcare, quite unlike disease care where acute injury or life-threatening disease may not provide options or even the opportunity to consider options. But understand the difference, and cultivate healthcare. For chronic problems, ask functional questions and consider all possible options for improving your body's function. Continue to fortify yourself to face a future of unknowns.

Congratulations on making it this far. You have graduated not only to an improved state of health but also to a new awareness of how you can create health and quality time. Your health plan contains the guidance for you to continue—for a lifetime.

It's simply a matter of shifting your attention from avoiding disease to creating health. Don't ignore disease. But focus on health.

Thank you for making a difference.

And please, tell your friends.

RESOURCES

To find an Applied Kinesiologist or for information about professional training to become one, contact the International College of Applied Kinesiology (ICAK):
www.icakusa.com
www.icak.com (outside the United States)
(913) 384-5336

To find a NeuroEmotional Technique (NET) practitioner, contact N.E.T., Incorporated:
www.netmindbody.com
1-800-434-3030 for additional referrals

To find a Sacro Occipital Technique (SOT) practitioner, contact the International Sacro Occipital Research Society:
www.sorsi.com
or the Sacro Occipital Technique Organization-USA:
www.soto-usa.org

To find a Doctor of Chiropractic, contact the American Chiropractic Association:
www.amerchiro.org
www.chiropractic.org (outside the United States)

To find an acupuncturist, contact the National Certification
Committee for Acupuncture and Oriental Medicine:
www.nccaom.org
(703) 548-9004

To find a holistic dentist, contact the Holistic Dental Association:
www.holisticdental.org
or the International Academy of Oral Medicine and Toxicology:
www.iaomt.org
(863) 420-6373
or Chirodontics.com:
www.chirodontics.com

To find a Functional Medicine Doctor, contact the Institute for
Functional Medicine:
www.functionalmedicine.org
1-800-228-0622

To find a Doctor of Naturopathy (ND), contact the American
Association of Naturopathic Physicians:
www.naturopathic.org

To find a Touch for Health practitioner, contact Touch for Health:
www.touch4health.com

To find a CranioSacral practitioner, contact the Upledger Institute:
www.upledger.com
1-800-233-5880

To find a doctor who specializes in environmentally sensitive
patients, contact Michael Lebowitz, D.C.:
www.MichaelLebowitzdc.com

For more information, including heart-rate monitors, diet and
nutritional supplements, and testing for food sensitivities, go to
Dr. Blaich's websites:
www.start2health.com
www.yourinnerpharmacy.com

NOTES

Chapter 1

1. World Health Organization, "The WHO Global Strategy on Diet, Physical Activity and Health: The Controversy on Sugar," *The Bulletin of the World Health Organization* 47, no. 2 (2004): 1.
2. World Health Organization, "Face to Face with Chronic Disease," 10 October 2005, http://www.who.int/features/2005/ chronic_diseases/en/; "Stop the Global Epidemic of Chronic Disease, 3 October 2005, http://www.who.int/mediacentre/news/ releases/2005/pr47/en/.
3. H. Holman, "Chronic Disease: The Need for a New Clinical Education," *The Journal of the American Medical Association* 292 (2004): 1057.
4. Johns Hopkins University, *Chronic Conditions: Making the Case for Ongoing Care.* Prepared by Partnerships for Solutions, Baltimore, Maryland, December 2002, 4.
5. J. P. Geyman, *Health Care in America: Can Our Ailing System Be Healed?* (Boston, Mass.: Butterworth-Heinemann, 2002).
6. A. Mokdad, J. Marks, D. Stroup, and J. Gerberding, "The Actual Causes of Death in the United States, 2000," *The Journal of the American Medical Association* 291 (2004): 1238–45.

7. T. Kottke, R. Stroebel, and R. Hoffman, "JNC 7—It's More Than High Blood Pressure," *The Journal of the American Medical Association* 289 (2003): 2574.
8. J. Crosby, American Osteopathic Association Daily Reports, archive for March 2005, http://www.do-online.org.

Chapter 2

1. A. J. Vita, R. B. Terry, H. B. Hubert, and J. F. Fries, "Aging Health Risks, and Cumulative Disability," *New England Journal of Medicine* 338 (1998): 1035–41.
2. L. Trupin, D. P. Rice, and W. Max, *Medical Expenditures for People with Disabilities in the United States, 1987* (Washington, D.C.: U.S. Department of Education, National Institute on Disability and Rehabilitation Research, 1995).
3. M. Mitka, "Jeremiah Stamler, MD: Researcher, Leader in Cardiovascular Disease Prevention," *The Journal of the American Medical Association* 292 (2004): 1941–43.
4. A. J. Vita, B. W. E. Wang, D. R. Ramey, J. D. Shettler, H. B. Hubert, and J. F. Fries, "Postponed Development of Disability in Elderly Runners," *Archives of Internal Medicine* 162 (2002): 2285–94.
5. J. F. Fries, "Aging, Natural Death, and the Compression of Morbidity," *New England Journal of Medicine* 303 (1980): 130–35.

Chapter 3

1. D. M. Eisenberg, "Trends in Alternative Medicine Use in the United States, (1990–1997)," *The Journal of the American Medical Association* 280, no. 18 (1998): 1569–75.

Chapter 4

1. H. Holman, "Chronic Disease: The Need for a New Clinical Education," *The Journal of the American Medical Association* 292 (2004): 1058.
2. H. D. Friedman, W. G. Gilliar, and J. H. Glassman, "Osteopathic Manipulative Medicine Approaches to the Primary Respiratory

Mechanism: A List of over 400 Papers Related to the Cranial Concept, and over 30 Books Explaining This Therapeutic Modality," San Francisco International Manual Medicine Society, 2000: 221–53; E. W. Retzlaff, and F. W. Mitchell, *The Cranium and Its Sutures: An Annotated Bibliography of over 250 Papers Relating to Cranial Manipulative Therapy* (Berlin: Springer-Verlag, 1987), 68; William G. Sutherland, *The Cranial Bowl* (Mankato, Minn.: privately published, 1939; reprint, The Osteopathic Cranial Association, 1948); Harold I. Magoun, *Osteopathy in the Cranial Field*, 3rd ed. (Meridian, Ohio: Sutherland Cranial Teaching Foundation, 1976); Viola M. Frymann, "A Study of the Rhythmic Motions of the Living Cranium," *The Journal of the American Osteopathic Association* 70, no. 9 (May 1971); E. W. Retzlaff et al., "Cranial Bone Mobility," *The Journal of the American Osteopathic Association* 74 (May 1975); D. Kostopoulos and G. Keramidas, "Changes in Magnitude of Relative Elongation of the Falx Cerebri during the Application of External Forces on the Frontal Bone of an Embalmed Cadaver," *Journal of Craniomandibular Practice* (January 1992); B. Libin, "Occlusal Changes Related to Cranial Bone Mobility," *International Journal of Orthodontics* 20, no. 1 (March 1982); M. Pick, "A Preliminary Single Case MRI Investigation into Maxillary Frontal-Parietal Manipulation and Its Short-Term Effect upon the Intercranial Structures on an Adult Human Brain," *Journal of Manipulative and Physiologic Therapeutics* 17, no. 3 (March/April 1994); J. Upledger and J. Vredevoogd, *Craniosacral Therapy* (Seattle: Eastland Press, 1983).

3. S. Oliveria et al., "Heartburn Risk Factors, Knowledge, and Prevention Strategies," *Archives of Internal Medicine* 159 (1999): 1592.

4. B. Braun, "Effects of Ankle Sprain in a General Clinic Population 6 to 18 Months after Medical Evaluation," *Archives of Family Medicine* 8 (March/April 1999): 143.

5. H. Kendall and F. Kendall, *Muscles, Testing and Function* (Baltimore, Md.: Williams and Wilkins, 1949).

6. G. Leisman, P. Shambaugh, and A. Ferentz, "Somatosensory Evoked Potential Changes during Muscle Testing," *International Journal of Neuroscience* 45 (1989): 143–51.

7. G. Leisman et al., "Electromyographic Effects of Fatigue and Task Repetition on the Validity of Estimates of Strong and Weak Muscles in Applied Kinesiology Muscle Testing Procedures," *Perceptual and Motor Skills* 80 (1995): 963–77.

8. R. Laheij et al., "Risk of Community-Acquired Pneumonia and Use of Gastric Acid-Suppressive Drugs," *The Journal of the American Medical Association* 292, no. 16 (2004): 1955–60.

9. L. Szarka and G. Locke, "Practical Pointers for Grappling with GERD," *Postgraduate Medicine* 105, no. 7 (1999): 88.

10. J. Putnam, "U.S. Food Supply Providing More Food and Calories," *Food Review* (United States Department of Agriculture, Economic Research Service) 22, no. 3 (September–December 1999), 11.

11. P. Maffetone, *In Fitness and in Health* (New York: David Barmore Productions, 1997).

12. W. Philpott and D. Kalita, *Brain Allergies, the Psychonutrient Connection* (New Canaan, Conn.: Keats Publishing, 1980).

Chapter 5

1. H. Selye, *The Stress of Life* (New York: McGraw-Hill, 1956).

2. Reduce Campaign, American Gastroenterological Association, http://www.2reduce.org/learn_more.html.

3. Ibid.

4. R. Callahan, *Five-Minute Phobia Cure* (Wilmington, Del.: Enterprise, 1985).

5. B. Moyers, *Healing and the Mind* (New York: Doubleday, 1993).

6. E. Sternberg, *The Balance Within* (New York: W. H. Freeman, 2001), 186.

7. J. Bland, *Genetic Nutritioneering* (Los Angeles: Keats, 1999); E. Roggero, E. Zuca, and F. Cavelli, "Gastric Mucosa-Associated Lymphoid Tissue Lymphomas: More Than a Fascinating Model," *Journal of the National Cancer Institute* 89 (1997): 1328–30.

Chapter 7

1. P. D'Adamo, *Eat Right for Your Type* (New York: G. P. Putnam's Sons, 1996).

2. E. D. Abravanel, *Dr. Abravanel's Body Type Diet and Lifetime Nutrition Plan* (New York: Bantam Books, 1999).
3. E. Lonn et al., "Effects of Long-term Vitamin E Supplementation on Cardiovascular Events and Cancer," *The Journal of the American Medical Association* 293 (March 16, 2005): 1338–47.

Epilogue

1. See chapter 1, note 1 above.
2. J. Astin, "Why Patients Use Alternative Medicine: Results of a National Study," *The Journal of the American Medical Association* 279, no. 19 (May 20, 1998): 1548–53.

Index

Beyond Words Publishing, Inc.

OUR CORPORATE MISSION
Inspire to Integrity

OUR DECLARED VALUES
We give to all of life as life has given us.
We honor all relationships.
Trust and stewardship are integral to fulfilling dreams.
Collaboration is essential to create miracles.
Creativity and aesthetics nourish the soul.
Unlimited thinking is fundamental.
Living your passion is vital.
Joy and humor open our hearts to growth.
It is important to remind ourselves of love.

To order or to request a catalog, contact
Beyond Words Publishing, Inc.
20827 N.W. Cornell Road, Suite 500
Hillsboro, OR 97124-9808
503-531-8700

You can also visit our website at *www.beyondword.com*
or e-mail us at *info@beyondword.com*.